Daddy King
and Me
Memories of the Forgotten Father of the Civil Rights Movement

DADDY KING
& ME

Memories of
the Forgotten Father of the
Civil Rights Movement

Murray M. Silver

CONTINENTAL SHELF PUBLISHING, LLC
SAVANNAH, GA

Continental Shelf Publishing, LLC • 4602 Sussex Place • Savannah, GA 31405 • www.CSPBooks.com

Photographs by Count Jackson, courtesy of the author.
Photo on page 122 by Donald Wickham.

Library of Congress Control Number: 2009928857

Silver, Murray M,
Daddy king and me. Memories of the forgotten father of the civil rights movement / -- 1st ed.
    p. cm.
  ISBN-13: 978-0-9822583-2-3 (pbk. : alk. paper)

Summary: "The author describes Martin Luther "Daddy" King's influence on the American political scene for over thirty years, and provides a first hand account of the ascent of many future politicians. The book spans 18 years, highlighting the relationship with "Daddy" King and his family."--Provided by publisher

Continental Shelf Publishing books are available at special quantity discounts for premiums, sales promotions, or use in corporate and community training programs. For more information, please contact: Sales@CSPBooks.com

Printed in Canada
100% PCW FSC certified paper
First Edition, July 2009

ACKNOWLEDGMENTS

The stories, quotes and conversations recounted in this book are based on my recollections, personal notes and journals, public statements and documents and, in some cases, review of published media reports.

From the start, I wanted to write this book myself, although I realized I wasn't a professional writer. I considered whether or not to write on my own rather than with a co-author. But because I wanted this to be a personal story, and fugit inreparabile tempus, I knew I had to write it myself.

After forty-four years, I retired from the private practice of law in 1997, moved from Atlanta, Georgia, where my family and I resided for thirty-seven years, to Hilton Head, South Carolina, and into relative obscurity. However, every time I met someone, the inevitable questions arise: Who are you? Where are you from? What did you do for a living? Merely acknowledging the fact that I knew the entire King family, from Daddy King, his illustrious son and daughter-in-law, through and including Daddy King's grandchildren, Andrew Young and family, Sam Caldwell and family, Jimmy Carter and family, Griffin Bell...prompted suggestion and recommendation, "You should write a book...this is American history...unique, intimate, revealing..."

This project has renewed my appreciation for the value of archival material. I have spent innumerable hours pouring over old letters and memos, saving much of it in files and boxes. My special thanks go to all those from whose letters I quote and reproduce.

I acknowledge with great love my parents of blessed memory, who were constant support and encouragement; my wife for over fifty years, Barbara; my sons, two best friends and critics, Murray, Jr. and Eric, their wives Cristina and Joan; the two doctors, brother Stanley and his wife Marcia; Bret and Cathy Seligman.

I am grateful to all those who offered encouragement, including our Atlanta neighbors and friends Jean Smith, Martha Plant, Sarah Bowles, Judge Charles A. Wofford, James M. Crews, and Bart Eason.

In addition, I thank Dr. Susan R. Groesbeck, Head of School, Hilton Head Preparatory School, Hilton Head, SC; Prof. Randy Stroud, School History Chair; Prof. Robert P. Sulek, Math Dept. Chair; Mrs. Margot Brown, Director of Institutional Advancement; Jordy Harris and Margaret Hancock. Each one, in their own way, offered me encouragement, consideration, friendship, and the opportunity to talk about and revisit the past.

Of course, I am responsible for the final contents of this book. I have earnestly tried to be frank and honest while honoring privacy, particularly that of my children, who are more important to me than I can describe here and have achieved so much in their lives. They, too, were deeply and permanently affected by all that happened herein.

With all of my trepidations about writing and with all of the complications inherent in looking back over a long and full life, writing this book has been a rigorous and absorbing exercise, one that I have enjoyed immensely. Throughout the book I hope I've given credit where it is due, and haven't neglected those to whom I owe so much. Needless to add, some names have been omitted. However, they remain in my heart.

Murray M. Silver
Hilton Head, SC
4 March 2009

CONTENTS

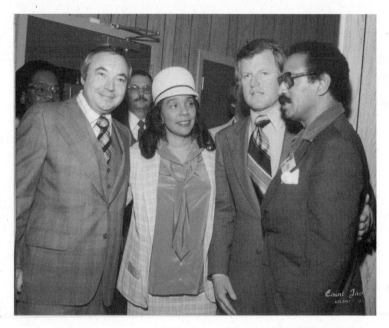

Murray Silver, Coretta Scott King, Senator Ted Kennedy in the foyer of of Ebenezer Baptist Church prior to the 1/15/1978 Annual Martin Luther King, Jr. commemorative service.

FOREWORD BY
MARTIN LUTHER KING III

In 1966, a genuine humanitarian named Murray M. Silver, Esq. began a friendship with my grandfather, the late Martin Luther King, Sr. that spanned a period of eighteen years. Mr. Silver's unique and historic story dedicated to honoring the memory of our "Daddy King" is filled with rare photographs and previously unpublished events involving several national leaders. "Daddy King and Me" is a visually descriptive and quick read that answers some provocative questions and will perhaps raise some additional ones.

Martin Luther King III
3 February 2009

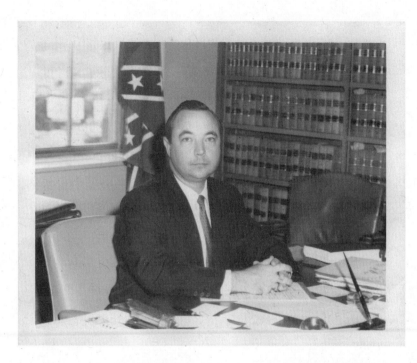

*Murray M. Silver, ESQ, General Counsel, GA Dept of Labor,
ESA, 1967*

A Most Necessary
Introduction

Several years ago, following my retirement from the practice of law, I was encouraged to write a book about a remarkable friendship with one of the most important men of the Twentieth Century, Martin Luther King, Sr., also known as Daddy King. It all began quite by accident and an incredible twist of fate.

It was the winter of 1966 when that fateful telephone call was received from the Judge of Superior Court in Camden County, Georgia. "Mister Silver, this is Judge Flexer. I'm calling you as a last resort. I need a lawyer with criminal experience to represent a black man accused of the murder of two prominent white men."

"Why me, Judge?"

"Frankly speaking, I've asked several other lawyers and they all refused, including Eugene Gadsden, the black lawyer in Savannah who is president of the NAACP. The problem is that this is a highly emotional case and the district attorney is going to seek the death penalty. How about it? I really need your help. And, oh yes, the county can probably pay you two hundred dollars to represent him. Please, I cannot accept no as an answer."

"Judge, I'll represent the man."

"Thank you. I'll never forget you for this."

The initial meeting with Robert Felton Moore in the cold, dilapidated jail remains a vivid memory: he sits alone, early twenties, tall, gaunt, scared, and beaten.

"Who are you?" Moore asks.

"A lawyer."

"I don't want no white lawyer. I want a black lawyer. What happened to the black lawyer from Savannah?"

"He refused the case. He said it was too much and too hot. The judge tried to get others, but everyone has turned him down. Looks like you're stuck with me."

Briefly stated, after a vigorous pursuit, the suspect was arrested, handcuffed and taken to the sheriff's office, interrogated for hours on end without benefit of counsel, threatened, beaten, and finally had the barrel of a loaded pistol pressed into his temple as the sheriff demanded, "If you don't tell us what you did to those two men, I'm gonna blow your goddam brains out!"

Needless to add, that prompted a confession which led to the discovery of the two partially clad bodies where they lay shot in the woods of Camden County.

The trial of Robert Felton Moore commenced on April 12, 1966. The entire community in southeast Georgia was outraged and emotions rose to a fevered pitch, prompting the suggestion that the trial was "an unnecessary expense...just hang the bastard." I was personally subjected to threats by phone and mail, culminating in the burning of a cross on the front lawn of my office in Brunswick. There was widespread publicity on radio and television, and newspapers as far away as *The Atlanta Journal Constitution.*

On the second day of the trial, a group of four black preachers from Atlanta made their way through a hostile all-white crowd surrounding the court house and entered the hot, humid, packed courtroom and found seats on the last row of benches. During the lunch break, I walked across the street and a few blocks to the Pure Oil station on Highway 17 for a Coca-Cola and a package of Lance peanut butter crackers. Upon my return to the court house, I was approached by the group of black preachers who told me that they had watched the morning session.

At that point, Rev. Martin Luther King, Jr. said to me, "It looks like you're really trying to help that man."

"That's my job, sir."

"I understand, but we've got to stop the killing. I'm trying to stop the killing."

"I understand, Reverend. But the police beat a confession out of this man and we've got to stop that, too."

Dr. King paused. "God knows your job is impossible, but we know—and He knows—that you are trying, really trying to help that man, and we thank you. Please, give us your card."

I reached into my wallet and withdrew my business card and handed it to Dr. King. We shook hands all around and I excused myself and turned to make my way through the crowd of angry faces toward the court house steps.

Dr. King stopped me. "You know, you are unusual," he said. "You march to the beat of a different drummer. May

Daddy King and Me

God continue to bless you and guide you in all that you do." Bernard Lee, Rev. Ralph Abernathy, and Rev. Fred C. Bennette, Jr. all nodded in agreement.

I was humbled by the experience, grateful for their appreciation, and thankful for the only kind words I received during the difficult trial.

Moore was convicted after a thirty-two minute deliberation by the jury, during which the jurors spent more time arguing over who should be the foreman than whether the defendant was innocent or guilty. He was sentenced to death in the electric chair on April 15, 1966, by Judge Winebert Dan Flexer. At that point I was released from further representation by the court, but I advised Judge Flexer that I would be handling the appeal.

"If so, it will be done without compensation by the county," Judge Flexer said. "We do not have the funds available."

"Judge, I told Solicitor General Jack Ballenger that if he used a coerced confession in evidence that I would fight him 'til the day I die."

"Then you're on your own," Judge Flexer said, and banged the gavel.

I handled all the appeals in Moore vs. State of Georgia, 222 Ga 748, 1966:
   • *Moore vs. Dutton, Warden, Ga 1967*
   • *Moore vs. Dutton, Warden, US District Court, S.D. of Ga, 1968*

- *Moore vs. Dutton, Warden, US Court of Appeals, 5ᵗʰ Cir., 1968*
- *Moore vs. Dutton, Warden, US District Court, S.D. of Ga, 1970*
- *Remanded to the US District Court, S.D. of Ga, 1970*

More than four years of the most emotional, gut wrenching appeals, at a personal cost of $12,000, the proceedings were so contentious that the U.S. District Court Judge Frank Scarlett threatened me with jail for contempt when I dared show up in his court a second time on an appeal that he plainly did not want to hear. I had no alternative but to consult with Scarlett's counterpart, Griffin Bell, the U.S. District Court Judge for the Northeastern District, Atlanta Division.

Bell was most supportive, and stated, "If you believe in your case, you must risk the possibility of being cited for contempt and incarcerated. Frank Scarlett is a tough old bird, but fair. One thing is for certain: Your profession owes you a tremendous debt of gratitude."

Bell's comments, especially the recognition of my sacrifice, caused me to shed tears. I went back into battle in Judge Scarlett's court with a renewed sense of purpose and prevailed, at least enough to get the case heard before the U.S. Court of Appeals.

On January 11, 1967, I was appointed General Counsel for the Georgia Department of Labor's Employment Security Agency by Sam Caldwell, Commissioner. My job—as the second highest legal ranking in the State of Georgia—was to ensure the fair and equal treatment of blacks seeking employment at the same time that Georgia had elected Lester Maddox our new governor, a segregationalist who was infamous for running off black patrons from his restaurant with an axe handle. Imagine my predicament when—just seven days after taking office—Dr. Martin Luther King, Jr. led a group of 35 black preachers and activists from his office on Auburn Avenue to the Labor Department Building a few blocks away, and requested a meeting with Commissioner Caldwell.

The Commissioner summoned me to his office. "There's a group of black preachers wanting to talk to me about something. Find out what they want."

It was my first official act as General Counsel to greet Dr. King and assure him that the new administration would see to it that all job applicants would be treated fairly without discrimination due to race, creed, color or gender. My pledge produced a low rumble of discontent among some of the assemblage. "You're saying nothing new," one of the protesters said, when Dr. King cut him off with a wave of his hand.

"I know this man," King said, pointing at me. "If Mr. Silver says it, I accept it, and gentlemen, we have no further business with regards to this matter." Rev. Bennette and Rev. Abernathy, whom I had met on the front lawn of the

---

Photos facing page
Top: *Silver delivering a speech in Gainesville, GA, sided by Sam Caldwell.*
Bottom: *Marguerite Schott, Mary Dabney, secretary to Commissioner, Sam Caldwell, Commissioner of Labor,Virginia Long-Caldwell's sister-,unkown, Danny Long. Back row: Fred Ray, Murray Silver, "Big" Lee Weir, National League Basebal Umpire; in Commissioner's office. Jan.1970*

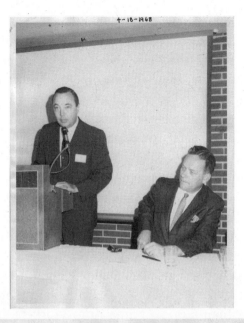

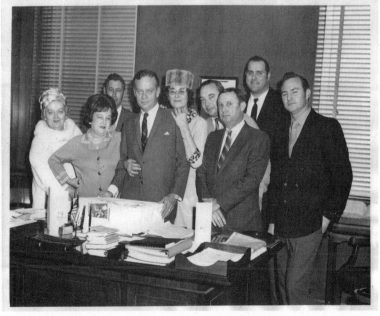

19

Camden County court house during the Moore trial, greeted me warmly and pledged their cooperation with the Labor Department. In the days ahead, Commissioner Caldwell and I prevailed upon Governor Maddox to hire blacks in government and it is a point of pride that the Maddox administration hired more black employees than any other administration before or since.

A few days following Dr. King's appearance at the Labor Department, Rev. Bennette invited me to lunch at The Varsity, the world famous drive-in across the interstate from Georgia Tech and home of the best hot dog on the planet. Rev. Bennette suggested that I take the time to meet Dr. Martin Luther King, Sr., as he, Leon Hall and Rev. Bernard Lee had discussed me with Daddy King, with reference to a wildcat strike at a Mansfield, Ohio plant that would idle the more than 6,000 Atlanta Auto Workers employed at the local General Motors plant, many of whom were black, and further deny them benefits, salary and unemployment compensation.

I thoroughly investigated the matter and worked around the clock to prepare necessary briefs to the Commissioner, filed a legal brief and opinion to the Georgia Supreme Court, which was accepted, published and enacted, even though Chief Justice Duckworth held that the employees were not entitled to unemployment compensation. Jubilant labor leaders descended upon Commissioner Caldwell, who introduced his General Counsel as "the man of the hour." We received congratulations from Walter Reuther, president of United Auto Workers, and the gratitude of thousands of auto workers and their families. Of all the notices we received, none was more gratifying than the acknowledgments from Dr. King.

The law was subsequently changed and remains Georgia law to this day.

Rev. Bennette made the appointment for me to meet Rev. King, Sr. at his office at Ebenezer Baptist Church on Auburn Avenue, a spiritual home to the residents of the "Sweet Auburn" community, where Daddy King had served as pastor since 1931. I can honestly say I was excited to meet this great man and being introduced to Daddy King by Rev. Bennette was a blessing. My first impression of Daddy King was that he was a huge man with a radiant smile, firm handshake; a most imposing figure. His desk was piled high with letters, books, bills, notes and the bible. The meeting began much like an interview: Daddy King inquired who I was, where I was born, educated, married, children, religion; how did I come to be in Atlanta, and the Labor Department? The conversation was casual, pleasant, friendly and relaxed. When we discovered that my father and Daddy King had been born in the same year, 1899, we formed an instant rapport. And, just as I had answered all of his personal questions, he—without being asked—told me about his marriage to Alberta on Thanksgiving Day, 1926, and his favorite reminiscences of his three children-- Willie Christine (Christine Farris), Alfred Daniel (AD) and Martin Luther, Jr.—all three born within their first four years of marriage.

I left our initial meeting impressed with Daddy King's keen mind, interest and kindness. Rev. Bennette subsequently pointed out that Daddy King and I "bonded" at this first meeting. I considered that event to have been so remarkable and important that I made a series of notes about our conversation that I preserved in a brown leather brief case, which I've added to over the years after other remarkable meetings. From that day forward I saw Daddy King frequently, and after I resigned as General Counsel on May 27, 1970, after more than three years of public service with distinction, and opened law offices in Colony Square on Peachtree at Fourteenth Street, I was in constant touch with Dad. Unquestionably, he was a giant of a man and one of my very favorite people of all time.

On December 7, 1970, the U.S. District Court for the Southern District of Georgia issued the order setting aside the death sentence of Robert Felton Moore and granting the writ of habeas corpus. The case was WON! After four long, hard years, the case which everyone in Georgia's legal system said had no chance to prevail had succeeded, and became one of the landmark cases—Georgia's Miranda case—in the process.

Thus begins the odyssey—an extended adventurous voyage.

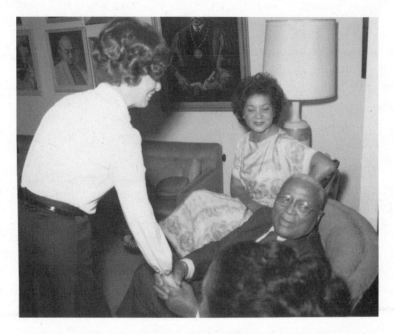

Barbara Silver greeting Daddy King at the King residence.
In the background is Alveda King Beal. Note the prominent
placement on their living room wall, of a portrait of Gandhi.

Chapter One

A Most Uncommon
Common Ground

From the beginning of our friendship, Daddy King wanted me to know a little bit about him and even more about Ebenezer Baptist Church. The church takes its name from the bible, "Then Samuel took a rock...and named it Ebenezer, for he said, 'This far the Lord has helped us.'" 1 Samuel 7:12. Ebenezer means "stone of help."

He was born Michael King on December 19, 1899, in Stockbridge, Georgia, to Delia and James King, the eldest son of nine children. The King family were sharecroppers but young Michael quit what amounted to slave labor when his father's boss threatened him after pointing out how his family was being mistreated. It was then that he decided he wanted to be a minister and more particularly wanted to fashion himself after ministers who preached racial equality. In 1918, he left Stockbridge for Atlanta, where his sister Woodie was boarding with Rev. Adam Daniel Williams, Pastor of Ebenezer since 1894. It was Pastor Williams who led the church through its developmental period, finally to the 407 Auburn Avenue location. It was this same Pastor Williams who encouraged Michael to finish his high school education and to become a preacher.

In 1926, Michael began his ministerial degree at Morehouse and on Thanksgiving Day married Pastor Williams' daughter Alberta, after eight years of courtship. Just past noon on January 15, 1929, a son was born to Michael and Alberta in an upstairs bedroom at 501 Auburn Avenue, one block from Ebenezer Church, in the midst of the neighborhood known as Sweet Auburn. A daughter, Willie Christine, followed in 1927, and a son, Alfred Daniel (AD), in 1930.

Following Rev. Williams' death in March 1931, Rev. King became pastor of Ebenezer. These were not easy times, the country in the midst of the Great Depression, and church finances were in dire straits. The three King children were sent to live with their grandparents. Rev. King organized the church's small membership and held fundraising drives, restoring Ebenezer to a strong financial basis. By 1934, Rev. King had become a widely respected leader in black Baptist circles and changed his name from Michael to Martin Luther King, reflecting his admiration for the German religious reformer. But it wasn't the sale of indulgences that kindled the fire of reformation in Daddy King; it was the need for an educated, politically active black ministry that turned the pulpit of Ebenezer into a bully pulpit of social reform. He led the fight for equal pay among Georgia teachers and also played an instrumental role in ending Jim Crow laws in the state, which had relegated blacks to a segregated subordinate state since the end of the Civil War. At the height of his political involvement, Daddy

King was a spearhead of the civil rights movement long before his illustrious son, rising to the head of the NAACP in Atlanta and the Civic & Political League.

During the course of our initial conversation many of the details were delivered casually and when it seemed Daddy King could not recall dates he paused, scratched his head and made notes on a pad in front of him. He took pride in accuracy.

I prefer to think of history as a chronological record of events, including an explanation of or commentary on those events. That part of my journey that I shared with Daddy King at our first meeting began in Savannah, Georgia, on December 23, 1953, three months following the birth of my oldest son and shortly after opening my first law office in the Savannah Bank Building, at the corner of Bryan and Bull streets, one block from City Hall. I recalled that it was a cold day, around 1 p.m., lunch time. Proceeding towards Morrison's Cafeteria, I witnessed the most upsetting event: a young black man being dragged by his heels, feet first, out of the cafeteria by several white men, and ordered never to return under threat of jail for trespass and causing a public disturbance. That man was Savannah native Hosea Williams, who later became one of Martin Luther King, Jr.'s lieutenants in the civil rights movement; that indelible impression of Hosea being rousted out of Morrison's remains with me to this day.

Daddy King interrupted me to interject, "Hosea Williams...I've known him since he moved to Atlanta...the Southern Christian Leadership Conference...had some problems with the NAACP...I recall he led the integration of the passenger train Nancy Hanks, that ran from Savannah to Atlanta, sometime around 1957...Hosea's slogan is

'Unbought and Unbossed.'"

I continued: "Many people regard Hosea as a trouble maker, but few of them realize that he is an educated man with a degree in Chemistry from Morris Brown and a Masters from Atlanta University. Many of these same people are unaware that Hosea enlisted in the army at the onset of World War II, and served in an all-black unit attached to General Patton's Third Army, where he was wounded in combat. I knew Hosea in the early Sixties, when he was vice president of the Savannah NAACP, under W.W. Law."

Dad was impressed with my knowledge of Hosea, unaware that I was aware of the fact that Hosea was with Martin when he was assassinated in Memphis. Thereafter, I frequently ran into Hosea as he established his "Feed the Hungry" program during the early Seventies, then entered politics as a Georgia State Representative, from 1974-85, as a member of Atlanta's council, from 1985-90, and as a Dekalb County Commissioner, from 1990-94.

There weren't many people in Hosea's circle who could get a rise out of him as I could whenever I reminded him of a time back in 1970, as my son and I were starting out in the concert business, and Hosea threatened to boycott one of our shows starring Billy Preston, unless we paid him for his "cooperation," which was Hosea's code word for promising to make sure that profits from such ventures would be redistributed among Atlanta's less fortunate.

(HISTORICAL NOTE: *In 1962, Martin Luther King, Jr. declared, "Savannah, Georgia, is the most integrated city south of the Mason-Dixon Line as a direct result of the leadership of Hosea Williams.")*

The single most important impression I want to leave

the reader with is that history has not paid Martin Luther King, Sr. his due. If the civil rights movement had a father, it was Martin Luther King, Sr., in the same way that he was father to his son: Daddy King trained, lectured and mentored Martin Luther King, Jr. In 1948, MLK Jr. became his father's associate pastor and he developed his ability as a speaker under his father's tutelage. Many folks will tell you: "If you ain't been prayed over by Daddy King, you ain't been prayed over!" And it is clear to me that the apple did not fall far from the tree.

(EDITORIAL NOTE: *It is particularly appropriate here—as the events I am about to reveal are not only true but previously undisclosed—to note that it would take me several hundred pages to completely describe my association of seventeen years with a man whom I believe was an incredibly great, outstanding human being. At this stage of my life I can only leave the vivid, lasting impressions that passing time cannot erase.*)

We talked about our families, especially our sons. Daddy King smiled as he recalled his children and often spoke of his devotion to his wife, "Bunch," which was his pet name for Alberta, shortened from "Honeybunch."

"Did you know that ML (as he referred to Martin Luther King, Jr.) learned to sing at an early age, from his mother? Bunch has been the choir director and organist at Ebenezer for as long as I've been pastor. That was something: ML had a good voice, accompanied his mother on organ. I smile every time I think about it. He was close to his mother. You know, we had it rough in the early days, the Depression days. ML was a child of the Depression."

"That's something we have in common," I interjected.

"Martin and I were both born in 1929, and both of us were born on the fifteenth day of the month; he in January, and me in October."

"ML did not want to become a minister," Daddy King continued, "and I did not insist that he become one. We never spoke about it. He did not decide to go into the ministry until his senior year at Morehouse. I think Dr. Mays had as much to do with ML's decision to enter the ministry as I did. Of course, ML came from a long line of preachers: my father was a preacher and so was my grandfather."

(HISTORICAL NOTE: *Dr. Benjamin Mays became president of Morehouse College in 1940, and was mentor to MLK, Jr. Mays was also a pastor of Shiloh Baptist Church. He gave the eulogy at Martin Jr.'s funeral in 1968.*)

One of the first questions Daddy King asked of me was whether I was a Democrat. My answer was a resounding "Yes," because my father was before me and I really did not have much choice: the Democrats were the power in Georgia, and any lawyer expecting to advance his career was going to have a hard time doing it if he was a Republican. Imagine my surprise to discover that Daddy King had been a lifelong Republican—that is, up until 1960.

"ML was arrested for trespassing during a sit-in in 1960, and jailed in Reidsville. This was during the presidential campaign and I was a Nixon supporter. But John F. Kennedy spoke about racial equality far more often than Richard Nixon, and when I became concerned for ML's safety in jail I put in a call to the Kennedy campaign. Bobby Kennedy secured ML's release and it was at that point that I switched parties. In fact, I promised to deliver ten million votes to JFK."

(HISTORICAL NOTE: *The defection of Daddy King to the Democrats led the way for millions of black Americans to follow. Traditionally, blacks were indebted to the party of Abraham Lincoln, U.S. Grant, and Dwight Eisenhower. The civil rights platform envisioned by Kennedy and enacted by Johnson won over the Kings.)*

Equal to my political leanings and perhaps more important to Daddy King was my religious affiliation. He was interested to learn that I was raised Jewish, even though my mother was a devout Irish Catholic; of the few white men in ML's inner circle, most of them were Jews. The subject prompted Daddy King to recall having attended the World Baptist Alliance in Berlin, Germany, in 1934, at a time when the host nation of the eleventh Olympic Games had begun constructing the Olympiastadion, slated for 1936. During this visit Daddy King became aware of a hostile environment toward Jews and blacks already in place and that its over-zealous nature was prevalent everywhere he went. Shortly after the conclusion of the World Baptist Alliance, Adolf Hitler made his dramatic appeal at a youth rally in Nuremberg, then turned his attention to the summer Olympics, which would've been a huge propaganda success had not the African-American sprinter Jesse Owens spoiled the party by winning four gold medals.

In addition to seeing Europe for the first time, Daddy King and a group of ministers visited the Holy Land, which not only formed a lasting impression but solidified his commitment to the ministry and formed a closer bond with Jews. He was fervently, deeply touched by the experience of seeing Jerusalem, as was recounted and reported in *The Atlanta Constitution*.

From May 17, 1954, when the Supreme Court of the United States ruled in Brown v. Board of Education that states could not segregate schoolchildren by race, until the end of the 1950's, more than one hundred homes, schools, and places of worship across the South exploded; the usual suspects were the Ku Klux Klan, neo-Nazis, and anti-Semites. In the early morning hours of Oct. 12, 1958, fifty sticks of dynamite tore through the side wall of The Temple, located in downtown Atlanta, where Rabbi Jacob Rothschild had led the congregation in support of the civil rights movement. Daddy King was the first to publicly denounce the bombing on television and in the newspapers, quickly followed by his son and his daughter-in-law. It may have not been the most popular thing to do, but it was the right thing to do, and when I asked Daddy King why he felt the urge to speak up in defense of the Jewish community he said, "The Lord is my light and my salvation. Whom then shall I fear? The Lord is the strength of my life. Of whom then shall I be afraid?"

A few weeks passed after my initial meeting with MLK, Sr. when Rev. Bennette called to tell me, "If you're comfortable with it, you can call Rev. King 'Dad.'" I was overcome with emotion, as this inclusion among the inner circle was totally unexpected. Few things could've made me happier, and was always careful to use the term of endearment with the proper dignity and respect.

Our next meeting began with a discussion about our fathers. Jim King had been an impoverished sharecropper with a strong work ethic, self discipline, dedication and determination. Daddy King's father was devoted to God and family, worked many jobs to help his parents, anything to get ahead. He was also keen on education.

I volunteered the fact that my father quit school in the third grade to shine shoes in an effort to help his family, who were poor immigrants living among people of every creed and color in Savannah; that, he too, was a dedicated family man, a proponent of education and having a strong work ethic. Conversation paused, Daddy King looked at me intently, nodding his head affirmatively.

Having mentioned that my father quit grade school in order to earn a living prompted Daddy King to admit that he was twenty years old before continuing his grade school education. Get the picture: a grown man, 20 years old, attending the fifth grade. It took him five years to graduate from Bryant Prep, from whence he entered Morehouse College in pursuit of a degree in theology. He graduated in 1930, one year after Martin Jr. and I were born.

"I made sure that my children got to school on time every morning, did their homework just as soon as they reached home in the afternoon, then did their chores," Dad said. "After supper they studied and before bed read and said prayers."

(EDITORIAL NOTE: *Christine King Farris does not remember growing up with her two brothers quite the same way. "Martin wasn't born a saint," she is fond of saying. "He got into his share of trouble...and he wasn't much for doing chores.")*

"It's evident that your devotion eventually paid huge dividends," I interjected.

He accepted the compliment, and for a moment turned almost boastful as he took great pride in relating, "As an adult I've never lived in a rented house, nor ridden too long in a car on which payment was due," he said, as if that bit of information might be useful. And it was, years later, when I assisted Dad in the purchase of a new automobile from Sam Troncalli at Troncalli Motors and advised Sam that financing would not be necessary.

Invariably, at some point in our conversations the preacher would come out, and I never came away from a meeting with Dad that he didn't take the opportunity to offer up a spiritual teaching. He was strong on self help, and often punctuated his advice with the promise that "The Lord helps those who help themselves." Unquestionably, he believed in the three R's: Respect for Self; Respect for Others; and Responsibility for Actions.

I remember a few years ago when Bill Cosby, comedian, actor, and activist challenged black Detroit to stop blaming white people for problems they could solve themselves, saying, "It's not what they are doing to us, but what we are not doing," and I remember Dad delivering those same lines. Cosby was hailed and often quoted, but Dad did not receive credit. And I remember fondly that many times during our conversations when he lapsed into preaching that old time religion of black pride and personal responsibility that Dad would pause dramatically, close his eyes and, as if thinking aloud, would say to me, "I think I'll preach on that Sunday morning."

There reached a point in our relationship, after he reached 80 years of age, where our conversations were much like his sermons: he spoke without notes, and delivered spontaneous comments that included everything from personal anecdotes about his family and friends to tongue in cheek harangues on the virtues of being Baptist.

I reminded him that on numerous occasions, members of my juries after trial would tell me that I missed my calling and should have been a Baptist preacher.

He had great expectations of Martin Luther King, III. Dad always spoke warmly of his namesake with a glint in his eyes. "Marty has an opportunity that very few men have in a lifetime; he's bright, has a nice personality, a good speaker...the big question is, does he have the desire to follow in his fathers' footsteps? It's a big decision to make." Then quoted Matthew 22:14: "Many are called, but few are chosen." Dad looked down and with a trace of smile, said to me, "We'll see, Counsel, we'll see."

When we talked family talk, Dad was quick to tell me about his firstborn, Christine, born in 1927. "She was always quiet, considerate, a good child, never sought the spotlight...a big sister to ML. In fact, she was the first of the kids to join church. ML came along later. They were happy children, stayed close to home. We lived in a segregated neighborhood, which was a problem for ML; he couldn't understand it, and told his mother so. Christine was a good reader, never gave us any trouble; a caring, loving child. At first she wanted to be a school teacher; I don't think she ever really considered doing anything else. She went to Spelman and then to Columbia University's Teacher's College. She was thirty years old before she was done, then came home to Atlanta and applied several times for positions with the local board of education and was turned down repeatedly. I don't know; maybe they were mad with me: I had a running battle with them for years over equal salaries for minority teachers. She was finally hired, but only after I complained to the mayor."

This was one of the most memorable events about Dad—his war with the Atlanta Board of Education over equal salaries—that was later confirmed to me as I stood in line at Morehouse College to pay final respects to him. There were two retired teachers standing in line with me, and when asked what their favorite memory of Dad was, they both stated emphatically, "His untiring efforts to aid and assist public school teachers in the early days, when we had no other help or support. He was our champion...for black and white...that, to us, was special. And we will never forget."

The second most important impression I want to leave the reader with is a clarification of the rift between Daddy King and his daughter-in-law, Coretta Scott, which, through the years, was roundly misunderstood even by members of the extended family, as a jostling for attention.

When ML met Coretta Scott in 1951 and the courting turned serious, Daddy King objected to the union, preferring that his son marry an "Atlanta woman." Coretta was from a tiny town in Alabama called Heiberger, southwest of Birmingham, between Tuscaloosa and Montgomery; residents of Alabama don't even know where it is. However ML was insistent, eventually convincing his father of his choice, and Daddy King performed the ceremony on June 18, 1953, at the Scott family home. Without a doubt, Dad quickly grew to love and respect his daughter-in-law. But there came a time, many years later, following ML's death and the establishment of the King Center in Atlanta, when it seemed to some that in trying to preserve ML's legacy not enough deference was paid to Daddy King and perhaps it was because of Coretta; that is simply not the case. Coretta would've been content to remain at home caring for her husband and raising children and grandchildren had fate not saddled her with the tremendous burden of carrying on her husband's work. She stepped up to the microphone only when it was thrust in her face, largely at the behest of Andy Young and other members of the movement who were not ready to take their places at the forefront and certainly not Martin's.

As a member of the founding board of directors of the Martin Luther King, Jr. Center for Non-Violent Social Change, I am often asked about this process whereby a quiet, unassuming preacher's wife became an icon of the twentieth century, and I am quick to point out that Coretta did not have anyone to model herself after. Jacqueline Kennedy did not go into politics following the assassination of John F. Kennedy; she ran and hid. There was no book written by a political widow for Coretta to take a page from. Who was she to emulate? Mary Lincoln? It wasn't that Coretta was ambitious; it was a matter of black America struggling to find its voice after The Voice had been silenced, and none of Martin's lieutenants could fill the bill in his same way, not without assuming the same risks. Andy Young came closest to replacing ML, but stepped away from the pulpit and sought the safety of public office where he was afforded a police protection that went nowhere near Martin Luther King, Jr. Coretta Scott King picked up a blood stained mantle and held it aloft for the world to see, and as her counsel and board member I saw it as my duty to ensure that her husband would not be forgotten, that his message of non-violence should not fade away.

During our many discussions over lunch at Paschal's

Restaurant, the traditional meeting place for black leaders in Atlanta since 1947, Daddy King and I discovered a number of unique similarities between the King and Silver families that some will dismiss as coincidence, that numerologists and astrologers might find interesting, but that I have always considered to be providential:

Martin Luther King, Sr. and my father Wolfe W. Silver were born in the same year, 1899. Martin Luther King, Jr. and I were born in Georgia in the same year, 1929, and on the same day of the month, the 15th; our first and middle names all contain six letters. Coretta Scott King and my wife Barbara were born on the same day, April 27th; both first names contain seven letters. Our first born, Martin Luther King III and Murray Mendel Silver, Jr. were born in Georgia in the same month, October.

It is further interesting to note that upon discovering Coretta and Barbara shared the same birthday that for many years the Kings and Silvers held a joint birthday party to honor both ladies, the first of these happy events being staged at the new Omni International Hotel in 1977, at which Daddy King presided over the festivities and blessed the honorees (photos of which appear throughout this text). And in November 1979, on the occasion of my oldest son's marriage, not only were Coretta and her children guests of honor, Daddy King made his last public appearance to give the newlyweds his blessing; that the Kings and Silvers were uniquely close in both our personal and professional lives cannot be overstated.

Of all the similarities between us the one aspect that has always meant the most to me was the message that ML and I learned at our fathers' knee. Daddy King often lectured his son on "Somebodiness": life is a blueprint, so

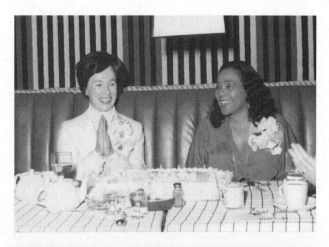

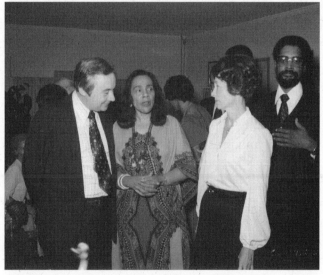

Joint birthday parties for Coretta Scott King and Barbara Silver. Above: 1977 at the Omni International Hotel. Below: 1978 at the King home.

to speak—a deep belief in your own dignity, your worth, what Dad called Somebodiness; you count, have worth, and your life has significance. In ML's speeches and writings the theme of Somebodiness comes through and is advanced. (Not surprisingly, Jesse Jackson used the chant, "I am somebody" to rally his supporters in later years.) My Daddy quit school in the third grade, shined shoes to help his family, taught himself to read, write and compute yet highly valued education, its importance and value. Prior to entering the University of Georgia School of Law, my Daddy lectured me, "You are going to be somebody...the first Silver to graduate from college...learn to express yourself truthfully, and treat others with dignity and respect." I like to think that ML and I became exceptional public speakers—often coming down on the same side of the same subjects—and became internationally known in our respective fields if for no other reason than we were raised by fathers who shared the same concept of Somebodiness.

On each and every occasion that I was privileged to be in Daddy King's company, I kept notes that I have preserved in a brown leather brief case, along with photographs and news clippings, just for that purpose. Realizing that he was serious-minded, studious and careful, Dad prided himself in promptness and courtesy; he always returned my telephone calls as soon as possible, saying, "If it's from you, I know it's important." In conversation, the nod of his head to whatever point I might be making mattered most to me. Unquestionably, he was a "Giant of a Man" and one of my very favorite people of all time.

At first, I must confess, I looked upon Daddy King as a father figure, to be listened to, respected and carefully consider his points of view. He was the exact same age as my father, who died in 1963. Then, as the days grew into weeks it was more like two old friends. On more than one occasion we talked like old friends, picking each other's minds, watching actions and reactions, swapping memories, thoughts, ideas, and suggestions. "Be who you are and say what you feel because those who mind don't matter and those who matter don't mind," was a point we both agreed on and discussed for hours.

Family matters, undoubtedly a favorite topic, showed Daddy King to be a strong, dedicated family man. There is no doubt that in his case it is around home and family that all great virtues are created, strengthened and maintained. Frequently, to the casual observer, it may have sounded as if our conversations were sprinkled with quotes from the Book of Proverbs, although in many cases what sounded like scripture were original with him.

Good fathers make good sons. My father was strong, a man of integrity, and if he told his four children not to do something, he didn't do it, either: he told us not to smoke or drink alcoholic beverages and although he was in the business of selling both, he did neither, nor, to the best of my knowledge, did any member of our family. My father was famous—at least around our house—for saying "Treat your family like friends and your friends like family. If you want to be respected, you must respect yourself."

How great an influence was Daddy King on ML? Tremendous, I say. Back in 1940, when ML was a mere lad of eleven years old, his father delivered a sermon to black clergy on the true mission of the church, in which he said,

"The spirit of the Lord is upon me, because he has anointed me to preach the gospel to the poor...in this we find we are able to do something about the broken-hearted, poor, unemployed, the captive, the blind, and the bruised." It is little wonder then that ML would preach the same message to a new generation when he launched the Poor People's Campaign of 1967, culminating in the March on Washington, in 1968. There can be no doubt that Dad was the inspiration for his son's ministry, and Martin often freely admitted that he followed closely in his father's footsteps.

I asked Dad on one occasion what was his proudest moment. His answer did not require careful consideration; he was at the ready with an answer: ML receiving the Nobel Peace Prize in 1964. Dad traveled with his son to Norway for the presentation. Tears streamed down his face as he gave thanks and recalled his family's humble beginnings in Stockbridge, Georgia, "that out of that tiny Georgia town, I'd been spared to see this and so much more."

Isn't it true that when a father gives something to his son, both smile and laugh, but when a son gives to his father, they both cry?

Perhaps it was Rev. Bennette who summarized my relationship with Daddy King best: we bonded.

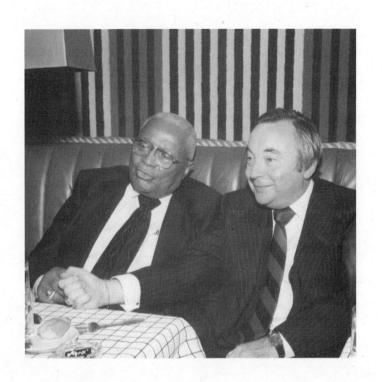

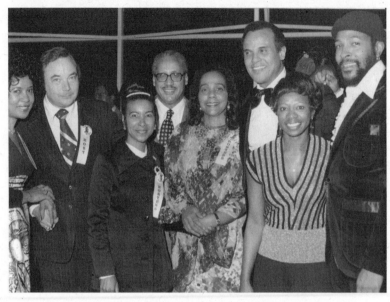

*Murray M. Silver, Xernona Clayton Brady
and Judge Paul L. Brady, Coretta Scott King,
Harry Belafonte, Mrs. Otis Redding, Marvin Gaye,
taken after the benefit concert to raise funds for the
building of the King Center. January 1975.*

Chapter Two

The Greatest
of All Time

I have always found footnote entries to some of history's great events to be of interest. I offer a few of my recollections of the events surrounding the death of Martin Luther King, Jr. in that same spirit:

On Saturday, March 30, 1968, Rev. Bennette called me at home to chat about current events. The purpose of his call was to find tickets for opening night of the Atlanta Braves baseball season on April 12, against the Cincinnati Reds. We talked about the team and its star players Henry and Tommie Aaron, Felipe Alou, Dusty Baker and Rico Carty. I had four dugout level season tickets in 1967; consequently Bennette thought I had connections.

During our discussion Bennette mentioned that ML was going to Memphis in support of the sanitation workers strike. ML had just returned to Atlanta from Memphis, where he led a march on their behalf that ended in violence, hundreds of arrests, and one death. ML's feeling was that he should not return, allow the situation to cool down, and then taking up the discussion again in a new voice that would "shed a different light on the matter." Bennette, for one, was definitely opposed to ML's returning to Memphis. Bennette had been ML's personal bodyguard and head of what amounted to security, both at home and on the road, at speeches and during marches. Bennette was hailed in the movement as "the man who picked up a live hand grenade" that had been thrown at ML and tossed it away seconds before exploding. Bennette gave me a telephone number where Dr. King could be reached and where he was meeting with his staff. Bennette cautioned me that the number should not be shared nor left casually laying about, for fear that the movement was being monitored by the FBI. I called Dr. King and had a brief conversation, wherein I echoed my conversation with Bennette that ML was not the best liked person in the United States and perhaps it would behoove him to postpone a return to Memphis. Dr. King's clear, unhesitating response was, "I appreciate your thoughts on the matter, however, this is something that I must do. I am not concerned about reports of possible harm while I am in Memphis...thank you for your consideration."

And that's the last thing that Martin Luther King, Jr. said to me.

Martin was killed April 4, 1968, while addressing a small crowd of people from the balcony of the Lorraine Motel in Memphis, shortly before he was to lead 1,300 sanitation workers in a march. A curfew was imposed on the city and 4,000 national guardsmen were called in to quell the riots that were expected but which never materialized. Bennette, who had remained in Atlanta rather than attend ML as his bodyguard, flew to Memphis with ML's sister

Christine King Farris to retrieve the body and accompany it to Atlanta, where the remains were entrusted to the Gus Thornhill Funeral Home. From that day forward Bennette never set foot on another airplane. "It just brings back those awful memories," he said. And from that day forward Bennette was never quite the same, pondering what might've been—or might not have-- had he been standing guard at the Lorraine Motel.

Many rumors of what might transpire in the hours and days following Martin's funeral in Atlanta had many residents fearing riots or some sort of reprisal from the black community, but there weren't any. I vividly recollect that the offices of Georgia government were closed and that many people who had no plans to join the thousands of mourners following behind Martin as he lead his last march hid behind closed doors with blinds drawn. I, along with Commissioner Caldwell and a few friends from the Labor Department, stood out front of our building and watched as the procession made its way past the state capitol. Thousands of people, wave after wave, mostly black faces clad in black clothing, and the thing I remember most was the awesome silence in spite of their great number, except for the random sob. Generations of families marched together, the very young as well as the very old, as if to say, "We shall not forget."

Another footnote that the reader may find interesting is that ML's funeral was held on April 11, the day before the Atlanta Braves opening day. Bill Bartholomay, the owner of the Braves, considered postponing opening day and called Daddy King for his opinion. "Martin would want the game to go on," Dad said...and viewed it from the owner's box the day after the funeral.

I visited Daddy King at his home in southwest Atlanta a few days after the funeral and shortly before we were to gather for Coretta's birthday. He was disconsolate, crestfallen, filled with grief, but still strong and resolute in his faith. He carried his burden with great dignity and bravery, "A spectacle unto the world, and to angels," as it is mentioned in 1 Corinthians.

"I need you to stay close to me now," Dad said to me, which was his endearing way of telling friends and loved ones to keep in touch regularly, but weeks passed before we were able to get together and spend time in conversation that did not revolve around ML's death. During the interim, however, I instructed Daddy King's housekeeper that I was available should he need me.

Following Martin's death, his brother AD, who was the pastor of a church in Lexington, Kentucky, returned home to Atlanta and was installed as co-pastor of Ebenezer alongside Dad. There was talk of his taking over the Southern Christian Leadership Conference and taking up his brother's mantle. He had, after all, traveled a twin path alongside his famous brother: a Baptist minister and civil rights activist, he was the pastor of a church near Birmingham, Alabama. AD made the news in 1963, when his house was bombed and outraged black citizens took to the streets seeking revenge. In an effort to calm the crowd, AD climbed atop a parked car and pleaded with the crowd not to resort to violence. "We have had enough problems tonight," he said. "If you're going to kill someone, then kill me. Stand up for your rights, but with nonviolence."

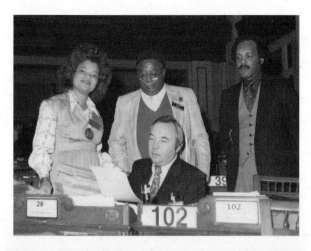

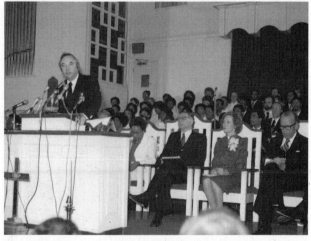

Top: Rep. Alveda King Beal, Fred C. Bennette, Jr, Murray Silver, unknown, in the House of Representatives after Ms. Beal's installation.

Bottom: Murray Silver addressing Ebenezer Baptist church congregation, 1/15/1979, during annual Martin Luther King, Jr., commemorative service. Seated L-R-Rabbi Arthur J. Lelyveld, Cleveland, Ohio; Mrs. Rosalyn Carter; Hugh M. Gloster, President, Morehouse College, 1967-87

Dad described his youngest son as an able preacher and concerned, loving pastor but did not seek the spotlight, even though he often appeared with ML at rallies in Atlanta and Birmingham. "As a young man, AD wasn't interested in school or church," Dad said. "He ran off and got married at seventeen and started a family. He got straight and decided to go to Morehouse...didn't graduate until he was almost thirty, like his big sister."

July 21, 1969, AD was found dead in his swimming pool at home; his drowning was ruled an accident. There was a routine police investigation. Under the circumstances, some believed then and continue to believe now that AD's drowning was not accidental and that he may have been murdered. The deaths of Dad's sons fifteen months apart would've devastated most men; Dad, although filled with grief, had reached the conclusion that nothing can bring back the hour passed; we will grieve not, rather find strength in what remains, in the faith that looks through death. The events of the past two years had added fifty to Daddy King.

AD was survived by his wife Naomi and five children. His oldest son "Ab," was dear friends with my oldest son, Murray Jr. His daughter Alveda King (Beal) became a member of the Georgia House of Representatives and followed the well-traveled family path as a minister, author, public speaker, ardent civil rights activist and founded King for America, Inc., in an effort to assist all people in enriching their lives spiritually, mentally and economically.

At the end of 1969, Bennette and Leon Hall advised me that Coretta was interested in establishing a memorial to her husband's memory and wanted to know if I would talk with her about the project. In addition to starting up a criminal law practice, I formed a company to promote rock concerts with my oldest son, a teenager with a love of music, and saw a way that Mrs. King might fund her venture through benefit concerts. Bennette, Leon Hall and I met with Mrs. King at the home she and ML had shared for many years on Sunset Avenue in southwest Atlanta, and where she continued to raise their four children. Joining us at that meeting was ML's sister Christine King Farris, who was the newly appointed treasurer of Coretta's foundation. This initial meeting of the board, such as it was, was held in Coretta's finished basement. Bennette quickly excused himself and went outside where he stood guard, as had been his habit as chief of security for ML all those years, intent that Mrs. King not suffer a similar fate to her husband.

In mentioning Leon Hall I would be remiss if I did not advise the reader of his position in the movement. He was only 21 years old at the time, but already a veteran on the scene for five years. He had dropped out of high school at 17 to join the marches in Selma and Montgomery, Alabama, where he first met Dr. King. Thereafter, Leon organized marches and coordinated student sit-ins at colleges throughout the South. Coretta thought that Leon would be instrumental in reaching out to the youth in establishing a living monument to her husband.

Coretta already had her eye on a site for the new center on Auburn Avenue, within easy walking distance of both ML's birthplace—which she intended to establish as a house museum—and Ebenezer Baptist Church. Conversation quickly turned to fundraising, with which she was totally inexperienced and unfamiliar, asking for suggestions. All eyes turned toward me.

"Mrs. King, I believe that we can call upon every black entertainer in America to join in a benefit concert with the proceeds going toward building the center. I have no doubt that many of them will donate their time and talent freely," I said.

"I think I could get my friend Aretha Franklin to appear," Leon chimed in.

And with that, there was a sudden joyful change in Coretta's expression. She took my hand in hers and said, "My goodness, that is a great idea. I hadn't thought of that. If you will assist me with this, I will be forever grateful."

My suggestion must've made quite an impression; it wasn't long before Daddy King called to thank me and to tell me of Coretta's excitement for the new project. Not that it was easy as running out and putting on a show; the old city auditorium was in disrepair and unsuitable for a stellar benefit fundraiser, and gaining the cooperation of talent management wasn't as easy as picking up the phone and asking stars to donate their time and talent.

In fact, the first concert we promoted did not occur until the summer of 1972, when I brought Richard Harris to Atlanta's brand new civic center. Harris was best known as the star of blockbuster movies such as *The Guns of Navarone, Mutiny on the Bounty, A Man Called Horse*, and best of all, King Arthur in Lerner and Lowe's *Camelot*. *Camelot* was also the beginning of an impressive recording career. In 1968, Harris had two gold albums, *MacArthur Park* and *A Tramp Shining*, and four years later included Atlanta in his first concert tour. That he was an unabashed follower of Martin Luther King, Jr. was no secret; meeting Coretta Scott King and Andrew Young backstage after the performance was "tantamount to meeting the queen;

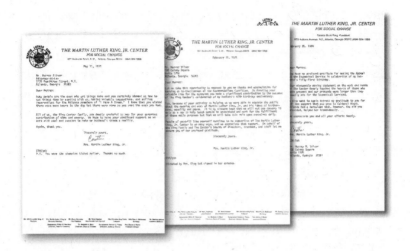

indeed, the first lady of the civil rights movement, as it were."

The following year Coretta introduced me to representatives of RCA Records who had taken it upon themselves to plan a major concert and record a live album at the Omni, with profits donated to the King Center. RCA had put together a stellar lineup: Wilson Pickett, Friends of Distinction, Jimmy Castor Bunch, Jose Feliciano, Linda Hopkins, Main Ingredient and comic Flip Wilson, and the best of each was included in a two-record set entitled, "Keep the Dream Alive." My job, as a member of the founding board of directors of the Center, was to coordinate the organization, development, presentation and ticket sales to the event. This concert was the inaugural event for the Omni, and we sold 20,000 tickets—every last seat in the house.

In 1976, I kicked off a series of concerts to benefit the building fund for the King Center. On January 15, we hosted a celebration of ML's birthday at which I served as chairman of the Accommodations Committee, arranging for all of the visiting celebrities and dignitaries, including Permanent Ambassador to the United Nations to Nigeria, Hon. Leslie Harriman. I keep among my personal letters the one from Coretta following this event in which she thanked me for my participation and for "having made a significant contribution to its success...on behalf of the King family and The Center...our profound gratitude."

On December 19, 1976, I staged an event starring Ben Vereen, who hosted a variety show on television and would in the following year have a starring role in *Roots*. The event was held in the ballroom of the Fairmont Colony Square Hotel, next door to my law office. The concert was originally intended to be a gift to my wife in celebration of our 25th wedding anniversary, and then the idea of holding a family reunion at the same time turned into an even larger family affair once we included Coretta, Daddy King, Jean and Andy Young, and a few hundred close friends. A few weeks later, on what would have been Martin Luther King, Jr.'s 48th birthday, we staged the first birthday benefit concert, starring O.C. Smith and the Emotions. Stevie Wonder headlined the birthday benefit at the Omni in 1979, and thereafter every other black singer on the planet lined up to take part in future celebrations. Management agencies that had previously refused or were slow to return my calls a few short years before were now calling me and offering us the best in the business.

But of all the events we ever staged, none can compare with the birthday benefit in 1975. That was the year that Harry Belafonte took the helm and, along with Sidney

Poitier, hosted a special viewing of their movie, *Buck and the Preacher*. Harry also prevailed upon Marvin Gaye to make a rare concert appearance. When Marvin sang, "Let's Get It On," let me tell you, the crowd went absolutely nuts. The task of master of ceremonies rather ceremoniously fell on me, and if I live to be 100, I will never forget standing at center stage with Harry and making an urgent plea for support for the King Center when suddenly we were interrupted by a roar from the crowd as Muhammad Ali walked onstage and snuck up behind us. Ali struck his famous pugilistic stance and squared off against Harry, who backed away, laughing.

"I got the fastest hands in the world," Ali said to Harry. "You wanna see how fast I can throw a punch?"

"Yes," Belafonte responded.

Ali stood motionless, the crowd in anxious anticipation. "Bam!" Ali shouted, without moving an inch. "Did you see that?"

"No," said Harry.

"You wanna see it again?" Ali asked, and the crowd screamed with laughter.

(EDITORIAL NOTE: *In 1967, Muhammad Ali had his license to box suspended and his title stripped by the New York State Athletic Commission in retribution for his refusal to be inducted in the army. He was allowed to box in 1970, making his comeback against Jerry Quarry in Atlanta, where Rep. Julian Bond had cleared the legal path and promoter Don King enlisted my help in drawing up the documents.*)

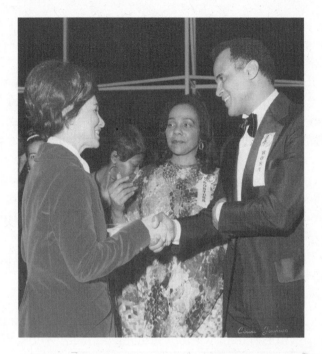

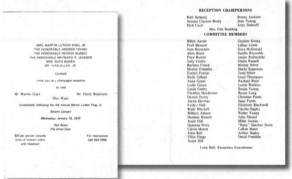

Top: Barbara Silver greeting Harry Belafonte,
with Coretta Scott King.
Bottom: Invitation to the Jan. 15, 1975 fundraiser concert

This event, more than any other, underscored the joy of the gains that had been made by the movement and more particularly the progress we made in funding the King Center. Perhaps there was no greater satisfaction to have received a letter of thanks from Mrs. King acknowledging that through the concert events we had raised more money than any other source, with the possible exception of Henry Ford II.

All in all, not bad for a poor country boy from Savannah.

Our families became good, close friends. For many years we gathered together to celebrate Coretta's and Barbara's birthday, April 27th. The first birthday parties were simple affairs in Daddy King's residence and Coretta's house on Sunset, and later moved to some of Atlanta's finest restaurants. Marty, Dexter, Yolanda (Yogi), Bernice (Bunny), Murray Jr, Eric, Christine and Isaac Farris, their son, Isaac Jr. and daughter Angela, Bennette...we were altogether. On each occasion, Atlanta's premier black photographer Count Jackson preserved the events in photographs which adorn this book.

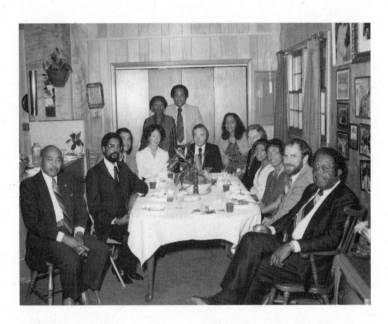

Standing: Christine King Farris and Isaac Newton Farris Seated L-R: unknown males, Barbara Silver, Murray M. Silver, Coretta Scott King, unknown females, Archer Smith, Rev. Ralph Abernathy

---

Opposite page -

Top: Murray Silver, Coretta Scott King at Atlanta Municipal Auditorium prior to a benefit concert featuring Gladys Knight and The Pips; Harry Belafonte.

Bottom: Murray Silver presenting Coretta Scott King with her portrait at a birthday celebration. Barbara Silver, Coretta Scott King, Bernice King, Murray Silver, Eric Silver, back to camera.

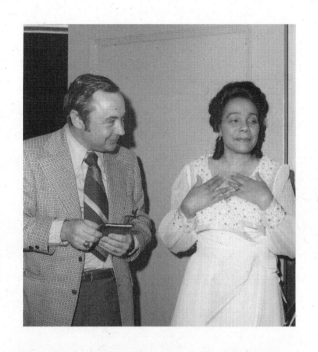

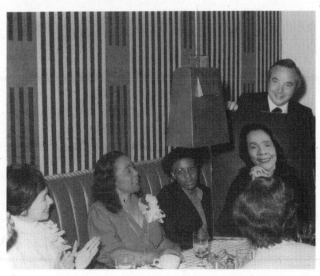

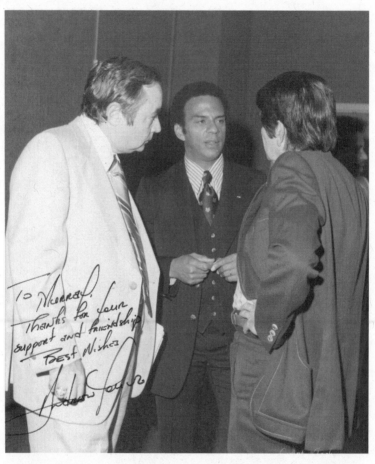

Murray Silver, Andrew Young, Truitt Crunkelton, AF of L,
fundraiser luncheon for Andrew Young Campaign, hosted by
Murray Silver, 1972.

Chapter Three

ENTER
ANDY YOUNG
AND
SAM NUNN

I was introduced to Rev. Andrew Young and his wife Jean by their close friend and associate Rev. Fred Bennette in 1969. Young was running for the U.S. House of Representatives Fifth District seat from Georgia against Rep. Fletcher Thompson. He did not win, but let it be known that he would try again. In the process of regrouping for his second attempt, Bennette came to me and suggested that Andy "needed a white face to help him and assist him in getting some sugar," which was Bennette's down-home way of referring to cold, hard cash. Bennette arranged the first meeting between me and Rev. Young, prior to which Bennette had taken me to school on Andy's background: born in New Orleans, he was three years younger than I; the son of a dentist and a school teacher, he entered the ministry in 1955, and moved to Marion, AL to pastor a church, where he met and married Jean Childs; by 1959, he had made black voter registration his mission, and moved to Atlanta in order to join the Southern Christian Leadership Conference (SCLC), and rose in the ranks to become its executive director in 1964; in this new role Andy became a close associate of Dr. King, Jr., and was a chief strategist and negotiator in their efforts in Alabama.

Upon meeting Rev. Young the first time I instantly liked him. He was all at once sincere and friendly, articulate and opinionated. And he wasted no time in repeating his purpose by echoing Bennette's suggestion that he was in need of sugar—white sugar, at that. I was candid with the reverend in advising him that if he thought it was tough passing around a collection plate in a small, poor black Baptist church that it was even tougher trying to mill white sugar for a black candidate. However, I thought that the answer to Andy's financial dilemma could be solved in the same way I intended to fund the building of the King Center, through a series of benefit concerts. It might be tough to get a $20 donation out of supporters, but it would be infinitely easier if we gave them something in return.

After conferring with my oldest son and partner in the concert promotion business, we decided to invite Bill Withers to headline the benefit concert to formally kick off Andy's second campaign for congress on May 24, 1972. Withers had two back-to-back #1 hits with "Ain't No Sunshine" and "Lean On Me," and was the hottest act in the nation. Harry Belafonte agreed to be my co-host and to assist me as emcee. The money that we raised that night was the single largest campaign contribution Andy received and catapulted him to victory; his re-elections in 1974 and '76 were infinitely easier.

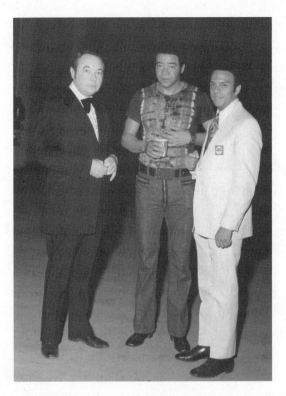

Murray Silver, Bill Withers and Andy Young backstage at the "Think Young" fundraiser concert for Young's campaign for Congress in 1972

Hosea Williams, a veteran civil rights activist and long-time acquaintance of Andy's could only sit back and marvel at his gains. "Andy Young can do more with white folk than a monkey can do with a peanut!" Hosea said to Bennette at one of our fundraisers. "That ain't Andy," Bennette corrected him. "That's Lawyer Silver."

In the process of managing Andy's campaign finances my wife Barbara and I and our sons became close personal

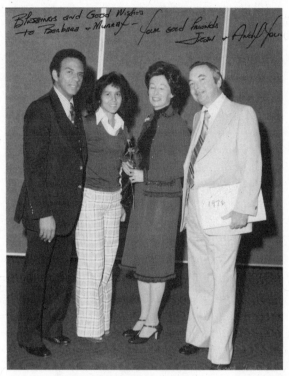

Andrew and Jean Young, Barbara and Murray M. Silver,
1972 luncheon for "Andrew Young for Congress."

friends with Jean and Andy Young and their children. Jean was a beautiful woman and a wonderful asset to her husband in all of his endeavors. She was an absolute blessing, a school teacher, religious, firm and friendly; Jean was every bit Andy's better half. Regardless of the occasion, the Youngs were always at the top of our guest list. And when congressional business took Andy to Washington far too often, we kept in close touch even if messages had to be relayed through Bennette, who was more reliable than Western Union and just as fast.

At the same time that Andy Young was gearing up for his campaign for congress in 1972, my dear friend Richard B. Russell, U.S. Senator from Georgia, died in office, causing a special election for his unexpired term ending Jan. 3, 1973. Governor Jimmy Carter appointed David Gambrell interim replacement, and the special election was slated for Nov. 7, 1972. It was around this time that I got a call from my old friend Sam Caldwell, who was still holding court as Georgia's Commissioner of Labor, confidentially advising me that Sam Nunn was interested in taking a run at Gambrell's position and the commissioner wanted to know if I would consider helping Nunn.

"Frankly speaking, Murray, Sam Nunn doesn't know any blacks," Commissioner Caldwell said. "And when he asked me who did I know that knew some, I, of course, told him that there is only one person in the state of Georgia who's on good terms with the black community and that he should call you. Which begs the question, are you already involved with Gambrell?"

"No," I replied. "I don't know Gambrell at all. He comes off somewhat as an elitist to me."

"Okay," the Commissioner said. "I'll tell Nunn to call you tomorrow."

I did not know Sam Nunn, but when he called me the following day he sounded like a long-lost friend when he invited me to meet him at his campaign headquarters in the Howard Johnson Motel on Interstate 85 at two o'clock the next day. Nunn impressed me with his candor, intelligence, quiet personality, and genuine desire to "meet some blacks." I began by suggesting he replicate Sam Caldwell's campaign all the way down to the color and typeface of his signage, as the commissioner had the best state-wide organization of any politician in Georgia, with Labor offices in almost every county, and that I had been Caldwell's General Counsel. I further suggested that he take a page from Andy Young's campaign by recording a song similar to the jingle, "Andy Young's gonna go to Washington," and suggested on the spot that he come up with something like, "Sam Nunn is tough, Sam Nunn is young, put Sam Nunn in Washington." It wasn't exactly Rogers and Hammerstein; nevertheless it made for a winning campaign theme song. Sam Nunn made careful note of my every suggestion, after which he asked me to pledge my support for his campaign, which I accepted.

The next day I phoned Daddy King and requested a meeting with him at Ebenezer, so that I could introduce the idea of gaining his support for Sam Nunn. I began by explaining to Dad that Nunn had been born in Macon, raised in Perry, was a family man and a good Christian. I told Dad that Sam was the nephew of long-time congressman Carl Vinson, another prominent Democrat, and that Vinson had always been sensitive to the plight of minorities; I saw no reason why Sam Nunn should be any different. After listening to my description of Sam Nunn, Dad shook his head and said, "Alright, let's go with him. You arrange the meeting, and I will talk to Ralph Abernathy and Coretta and one or two others."

Once Daddy King had assembled the most prominent black leaders in America, I personally arranged for Sam Nunn to be introduced to them at a private meeting, after which we embarked on a vigorous campaign to defeat David

Gambrell in the Democratic primary and won. Our next opponent in the general election was U.S. Representative Fletcher Thompson, whom Andy Young had replaced, and we won.

On Feb. 16, 1973, shortly after the new congress had been sworn in, I received a letter from Senator Nunn on his new stationery:

"During the first weeks of the 93rd Congress, I have often thought of the many individuals in Georgia whose hard work resulted in my assuming this responsible position of trust.

"I have a deep sense of gratitude to the people of Georgia for bestowing this high honor on me, and to you, personally, for your efforts to insure our success on November 7. Your personal dedication to my campaign contributed significantly to the outcome, and I will always be grateful for your friendship and support."

Following a few personal remarks, the letter concluded, "Thanks for 'Getting Tough in Georgia' and 'Putting Sam Nunn in Washington.'"

Signed, Sincerely, "Sam."

And now you know the rest of the story.

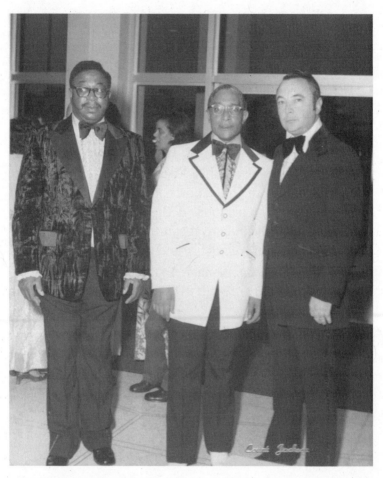

Fred C. Bennette, Rep E. J. Shepherd, Murray M. Silver. 1975

Chapter Four

I
CANNOT HATE
ANY MAN

There is an age-old legal maxim that I used many times in counseling clients and instructing witnesses: Always tell the truth, and then you will not have to remember what you said. Keeping that in mind, I record the following events with the utmost accuracy, published here for the first time:

Throughout all the years of our association, Daddy King frequently called upon me to represent indigent clients as a personal favor to him. Typically the client was a member of Ebenezer or a resident of the Sweet Auburn community and Dad knew the family, realized they were unable to pay for legal services, and prevailed upon me to lend a hand. The call usually came at night, at home, at the last hour: "Counsel, this is Dad. I hate to bother you this late, but Mrs. Taylor just called to tell me her son has to be in Judge

Wofford's court tomorrow, to stand trial for burglary. I know the family; they cannot afford to hire a lawyer...can you help them?"

I never turned him down.

"Thank you, Counsel. Next time I'll try to send you one who can pay."

There was always a "next time," but I never got paid.

Then came the call from Daddy King inviting me to attend services at his beloved Ebenezer, on Sunday, June 30, 1974. He set aside this day to formally recognize me for my many kindnesses and generosity in helping others, coming on the heels of having paid for repairs to Ebenezer's air conditioning system in the middle of an unusually warm Atlanta summer.

I drove from my residence in the Breckenridge community in Northeast Atlanta via Piedmont Avenue and was three blocks from the church on Auburn Avenue, listening to WSB radio, when John Pruitt broke in to announce there had been a shooting at Ebenezer. I arrived just as the emergency medical technicians were removing two bodies from the sanctuary and stared in disbelief. Three members of the church choir rushed over to tell me that Mama King had been shot while seated at the organ preparing for services. "A black man, a brother man, jumped up and hollered, 'I'm tired of all this! I'm takin' over!' and started shooting with two pistols," one of the choir members said, then broke down and cried before saying anything more.

The gunman had also shot and killed Deacon Edward Boykin, then sprayed the congregation with bullets, striking at least one other person. Two Atlanta police officers recognized me, came over and told me that Mrs. King appeared to be in critical condition. As the ambulance sped away, I went inside the church to find Dad—who had been waiting for me in his office rather than inside the sanctuary when the shooting occurred-- surrounded by church members. He sat in stunned silence, his face almost ashen, eyes closed, rocking back and forth in the embrace of his extended family.

On July 3, I sat with the King family as Dr. Sandy Ray, Pastor of Cornerstone Baptist Church in Brooklyn, NY, and Rev. LV Booth from Cincinnati's Zion Baptist Church officiated at the funeral. Mrs. King, dressed in a pale pink dress, reposed in a white casket placed in front of the altar only a few feet from the organ where she was seated when the gunman took her life.

Daddy King rose slowly to his feet looking as though the weight of the entire world was on his broad shoulders, searched the faces of his family, and ascended to the pulpit. He spoke slowly, barely audibly at first, and then gained strength as he took control, that deep voice resonating throughout the sanctuary just as it had on so many prior occasions. He praised Alberta's kindness, her love of family, and devotion to their church. "Her ways were ways of pleasantness, all her paths were peace."

At that point, a change swept over him, the memories of the tragic losses of his sons coming in waves. He did not break and he did not waver; he became defiant, as if provoked. "I'm not gonna quit and I'm not gonna be stopped!" he shouted, pointing to a place where the gunman had stood a few short days before. "We've got to carry on!"

And, as the congregation erupted in applause, Dad stepped down from the pulpit, approached the closed casket, placed his hand on it and gently completed his eulogy: "So, Bunch, I'm coming on up home. I'll be home almost anytime now."

The congregation gasped, amid tears. In all my years I have seldom seen a greater outpouring of public grief or empathy.

I did not hear from Daddy King for a few weeks following his wife's funeral, and then one day he called me at my office. I recall it verbatim:

"Counsel, this is Dad. How are you?"

"Dad, I'm okay, better now that I've heard from you. I hope you are feeling better."

"Yes, with the Lord's blessing, I'll make it. Can I ask you a favor?"

"Anything, you know that."

After a long pause, Daddy King asked me, "Can you arrange for me to visit the man that killed Alberta?"

After a long pause on my end, I replied, "Why, Dad?"

"I just want to look him in the eye."

It was—under these circumstances—a rather strange request, but I did not press Dad for details. I promptly put in a call to the High Sheriff Leroy Stynchcombe, whom I had known for the five years I had been in private practice, and asked for his permission to arrange a meeting between Rev. King and Marcus Wayne Chenault, who had admitted his crime with a rare enthusiasm.

"I've known Reverend King most of my life and consider him a friend," the sheriff said. "He sure has had a terrible time. But what I want to know is why does he want to do this?"

"Dad says he wants to look him in the eye," I said, without further embellishment.

"And you will accompany him and remain with him at all times?"

"Yes, sir."

"I don't want any publicity, do you understand?" the sheriff said. "I want your guarantee that there will be no television cameras, no newspaper reporters...I don't need publicity. You understand?"

"Sheriff, I give you my word: there will be nobody but Dad and me—no cameras, recording devices, nothing...it shouldn't take longer than ten minutes."

"Alright, then, I'll call the jailor and make arrangements for you to come in the rear entrance where we bring in prisoners. When do you want to come?"

"As soon as possible," I said, reflexively.

"Give me two hours," the sheriff said.

I called Dad immediately and told him that I would pick him up at his home at 3:30 pm. Upon my arrival I found him waiting in his living room, dressed in a grey suit and tie. "Thank you so much for doing this, Counsel," he said.

"I'm ready if you are," I said, "but I wish you would rethink this."

"No, I've made up my mind; I just want to look this man in the eye and ask him one question: Why did you do this?"

The ride from Daddy King's home to the Fulton County Jail took thirty minutes, during which time I mulled over what possible good could come from this confrontation. I feared for Dad's safety and for his mental and emotional welfare. In all my years practicing criminal law, I never encountered a family member of a murder victim who was so intent upon looking into the eyes of their loved one's killer. But for thirty minutes we maintained a dreadful silence.

Chief among my concerns was that Chenault was not in his right mind. The act certainly speaks for itself, but at his arraignment Chenault appeared defiant, calling himself Servant Jacob, and declared that he was sent here on a purpose and that it was only partially accomplished. He alternately referred to himself as a Hebrew and a Muslim, that he considered all ministers of the gospel to be liars and thieves, and that his mission was to rid the world of their influence. But my greatest concern was that Chenault had stated his purpose in going to Ebenezer on that tragic day was to kill Daddy King, and I feared the scene that might ensue once the two men came face to face even though they would be separated by iron bars. Investigators told me that they had found in Chenault's apartment a hit list with ten names; Rev. Martin Luther King, Sr. was at the top of the list.

Arriving at the jail we proceeded to the rear entrance where prisoners are processed. The jailor was waiting for us, swinging open the screen meshed steel doors; a most sobering reception. We were ushered into the cell block holding area where attorneys are permitted to visit clients, a place I had been too many times and yet never grew accustomed.

Chenault was brought down to the holding area and placed in the cell. His short, chunky stature was swallowed up by the day-glo orange prison garb. I entered first and stood at the entrance to the visitor's side of the cell, Dad stood to my left, slightly behind me. We were separated from Chenault by a partition of steel bars. No one else was present; just we three.

I studied Chenault carefully as he settled in a chair. He did not move or make any sign of recognition, looked directly at us.

Dad peered at Chenault silently for a few moments, balancing his massive weight evenly on both feet, adjusted his eye glasses and then in a clear, level tone asked him, "Do you know who I am?"

"Yes," Chenault replied.

"Why did you do this terrible thing?"

Chenault arose, stood erect, and erupted, "I hated her and I killed her; I hate you, and if I could have, I would've killed you, you dirty bastard. All Christians are my enemies!"

Dad rocked back on his heels as though he had been punched in the face. I grabbed his arm to lend support and was so upset by Chenault's threat that tears of anger and frustration welled up in my eyes. I pulled Dad out of the cell and toward the exit. "I hate this son-of-a-bitch," I said to Dad.

He placed his right hand on my shoulder and without hesitating uttered the words which will always be remembered and associated with him: "Counsel, I cannot hate any man."

I was stunned by his compassion and silenced by his conviction. I wiped away the tears, took his arm and walked to my car. The drive to his home was spent in utter silence. Dad sat erect but with an expression of unbearable sorrow, arms at his side as if too weary to carry. When we arrived he got out of the vehicle slowly, placing his hand on the hood for support, and then walked to the front door where his housekeeper greeted us. I accompanied him to his bedroom where I helped him undress and get into bed; he could not lift his legs. I stayed with him a while, sensing that he had something to say.

"Counsel, this is one of the most memorable events of my lifetime. I will never forget it, and I can only say thank you."

My heart was heavy and I wished that there was something I could do to help ease his burden. He closed his eyes and I took my leave, every detail of that afternoon firmly etched in memory.

In the days immediately following the confrontation at the county jail, I was contacted by agents of the FBI and interviewed. They were as curious about what had transpired when Daddy King met Chenault as I was interested in what their investigation had revealed. Special agents of the FBI do not make a habit of commenting on their findings, but when I related my first impressions of the culprit, that he was a Muslim; that he hated Christians in general and the Kings in particular; and that he was a terrorist, I got no argument from them. The agents acknowledged the information we had received that a hit list of ten black religious and civil rights leaders had been found in Chenault's apartment and that the name at the top of the list was Martin Luther King, Sr., but my questions as to Chenault's purpose and motive went unanswered. Weeks later, at Daddy King's behest, I made a formal inquiry into the matter and received a written response from the FBI headquarters in Washington that the case was sealed.

A year to the day following the death of Mama King, Daddy King resigned as pastor of Ebenezer. He had talked to me often about the decision and when it should come, but decided that there wasn't much to say after delivering the eulogies of his wife and only sons, and elected not to return for his 45th year of service.

We could not let the occasion go unnoticed. A group of us organized a retirement banquet, black tie, invitation only, on August 1, 1975, which I was privileged to attend with my wife and Coretta Scott King. Other than the day I married and the occasions of my sons' weddings, I can't remember putting on a tuxedo for too many other celebrations; we were not a country club crowd, but after all he had endured we thought that the least we could do for Daddy King was send him into retirement in style. My favorite memory of that evening was sharing memories of that time in 1969 when Rev. and Mrs. King were honored as "The Daddy and Mama of the Civil Rights Movement" with my dear friend Fred Bennette.

And I pause here to ask the reader one question:

Does a reader hereof know or have heard tell of any prominent person who suffered equal or greater losses by violence than Daddy King?

(EDITORIAL NOTE: *After trial in the Superior Court of Fulton County, the Hon. Luther Alverson presiding, the jury sentenced Marcus Wayne Chenault to Death on both counts of Murder of Alberta King and Deacon Edward Boykin, plus ten years in the penitentiary for aggravated assault, to run consecutive with the death* sentence. *He was placed on death row. Chenault appealed to the Supreme Court of Georgia, 234 Ga. 216, 1975, on the grounds that he was innocent by reason of insanity. The judgment of the lower court was affirmed. Chenault followed with other appeals. In 1995, after the US District Court upheld the sentence, a deal was struck between the defendant's attorneys and District Attorney Lewis Slaton, who agreed to Chenault being re-sentenced to life in prison in exchange for a cessation of the appellate process. In reaching this compromise, Slaton acknowledged Daddy King's opposition to the death penalty—even in the case of his own wife's murderer—as having major weight on his decision. Chenault died in prison of natural causes on September 4, 1995.)*

Chapter Five

AGAIN,
ON DOWN THE ROAD:
GRIFFIN BELL

As 1975 drew to a close, Jimmy Carter was completing his term as Georgia's 76th governor. Andrew Young called to invite me to attend what he referred to as a meeting of a few folks to talk about Carter's run for president.

"President of what?" I responded.

I had met Carter in 1966 as a Senator from Georgia's 14th district. He showed up uninvited at Sam Caldwell's annual "Wild Feast" banquet, at which the Commissioner of Labor feted his powerful friends, and hung around the entrance until I brought him to the Commissioner's attention. "Do you want me to invite him inside?" I asked Sam. "He's a state senator from Plains, yeah, sure," Sam said. And so I approached Senator Carter and invited him to join us.

My first impression of Carter was the antithesis of the classic Georgia politician in the Talmadge tradition: bold, assertive, boisterous, loud, a man of the people. Jimmy was quiet, unassuming, and had a soft, limp-wristed handshake. Sam Caldwell laughed like hell when I described Carter as such.

But here he was eight years later and a soon-to-be former governor intending to enter the Democratic presidential primaries, where he was roundly considered by political pundits to have little or no chance against household names like George McGovern and Ted Kennedy. Florida Gov. Reuben Askew and Henry Jackson, the Senator from Washington, DC, had greater name recognition than the peanut farmer from Georgia, who had been soundly defeated in his first attempt to become governor by an avowed racist restaurateur with no political experience. Even then, I sent my oldest son to work for Carl Sanders in an effort to defeat Carter in his second attempt. However, after being massaged by Andy Young and Fred Bennette, I agreed to support Carter in his bid for the presidency, actively campaigned for him, raised money, and chauffeured Rev. Bennette all over the state to rally black politicians and preachers. Honestly, I never ate so much fried chicken in all my life.

On June 19, 1976, Barbara and I attended the biggest and most successful fundraiser for Carter, hosted by my good friend and Colony Square landlord, Jim Cushman. I paid a record price for a Tommy Nobis Atlanta Falcons football jersey that had been donated to a celebrity auction, and received a beautiful autographed photo from Carter's #2 son, Chip, in thanks for our support.

Any politician looking to curry the favor of black voters in the Seventies could be expected to show up at Daddy King's door at some point in their campaign and Jimmy Carter was no exception. However, Dad's contributions to

Carter's fledgling campaign are not recorded nor does he receive the proper consideration he deserves. Dad played a notable role in getting Carter elected president. After making a splash in the Iowa caucus and the primaries in Florida and New Hampshire, liberal Democrats launched an ABC movement—"Anybody But Carter"—in an attempt to head off the nomination of the upstart peanut farmer. In staving off this attack, Carter resorted to Daddy King, who had supported Gov. Carter's efforts to end segregation and to end voting restrictions that had historically disenfranchised poor blacks. When northern liberals tried to whitewash Jimmy Carter as a racist, Jimmy countered by throwing his arms around Daddy King in a photograph that was picked up by every newspaper, magazine and television network in America. Daddy King was interviewed endlessly by these same news outlets, and the issue of Carter's political correctness was ended in his favor.

It must be stated as clearly and as concisely as possible: Certainly the single most instrumental and influential individual in building a coalition of black preachers in support of Carter was Rev. Martin Luther King, Sr.

Carter was elected.

Daddy King delivered the invocation at the 1976 and 1980 Democratic National Conventions.

On October 1, 1976, Andrew Young announced his intention to be re-elected to Congress; it was never really in doubt, as he was just getting his feet wet by completing his first term. Rev. Bennette sounded the clarion call; the Silvers responded. On October 23, my wife and I hosted a luncheon to raise funds that was well attended by many of our friends in the Labor movement. Herb Mabry and Herb Green, leaders of the United Automobile Workers (UAW), were present and pledged the support of their respective unions, representing more than 50,000 members. The "Two Herbs" and I had been political allies since Sam Caldwell's election in 1967. In recognition, Barbara and I were seated at the table next to the honoree and his wife, Jean. I addressed the gathering as host and master of ceremonies and recognized long-time Democratic Party leader Marguerite Ewing Schott, EL Abercrombie of the Laundry and Dye Workers Union, and Ted Clark. I keep in my scrapbook the letter I received from Andy following this event, dated October 25, in which he wrote: "Your continuing financial and moral support mean more than words can express..."

Andrew Young was re-elected.

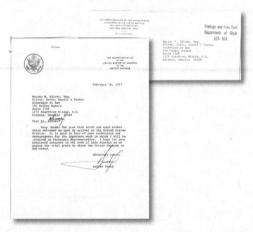

James Earl "Jimmy" Carter, Jr. was elected 39th President of the United States and was sworn into office on Thursday, January 20, 1977; the day began in a most symbolic manner: As Carter assumed the power, there was

Daddy King, evoking memories of his son delivering the "I Have a Dream" speech on the steps of the Lincoln Memorial. It was a clear, crisp day when Carter began his celebratory stroll down Pennsylvania Avenue, hand in hand with his wife Rosalynn, a most dramatic and truly memorable scene; the walk from the Capitol to the White House took forty minutes to cover the mile-and-a-half distance, departing from the traditional limousine ride.

We received an engraved invitation to attend Carter's inauguration. In addition, we were invited to a slew of A-list social gatherings and presidential balls. The historic Mayflower Hotel was our residence for four days, as it was Coretta's preference, and she wanted us to be near her. There we were, Coretta, Daddy King, Rev. Bennette, and Dr. Bernard Bridges, the King family personal physician, and a fabulous time was had by all. I never saw so many folks from Georgia in the nation's capitol, never heard so many "Hi y'all" in DC, either before or since.

One of Jimmy Carter's first appointments was Griffin Bell as his attorney general. I had known Griffin since 1958, when we were introduced by S. Ernest Vandiver, during his campaign for governor of Georgia. My dear friend and political mentor Sol Kaminsky, the renowned car dealer from Savannah, was one of Vandiver's chief fundraisers and solicited the Silvers' help, knowing that my father, the legendary pool room proprietor and restaurateur "Bo Peep" was a staunch Democrat and a major contributor to previous gubernatorial campaigns, and suggested that I get into politics. By that time I had only been practicing law for five years, and it was practically impossible to further a professional career in those days without political clout.

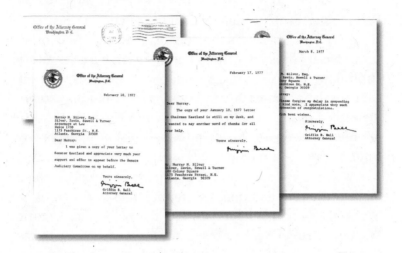

Four of us—Sol, Vandiver, Griffin Bell and I-- met in a suite at the DeSoto Hotel on Liberty Street in Savannah, across the street from Sol's office at his Pontiac and Cadillac dealership. Sol laid out five thousand dollars on the table and Ernie's eyes grew as round as moon pies; counted it, hugged us, and thanked us repeatedly for the largest contribution he had ever received.

Vandiver was elected governor of Georgia and served from 1958 until 1961. Sol Kaminsky was generously repaid as the official supplier of automobiles to the Georgia State Patrol; Griffin Bell was appointed Vandiver's chief of staff; Murray M. Silver, Esq. was named an honorary Lt. Colonel and received a Governor's Staff automobile license plate, which came in handy whenever I wanted to go to a University of Georgia football game and circumvent the traffic.

Let me remind my reader that this was the same Griffin Bell mentioned in the Introduction, the judge of the US Court of Appeals, Fifth Circuit, Atlanta, who once upon a time offered me wise counsel and a comradely consideration during the epic battle on behalf of Robert Felton Moore. It was Griffin Bell who encouraged me to confront his counterpart Frank Scarlett, US District Court Judge for the Southern District of Georgia, who had threatened me with jail for contempt of court in pressing Moore's case. Bell's even handed administration of justice guided me through the most perilous time in my legal career. His final words of advice echo in my mind even now: "If you believe in your case, that you are right in your legal position, you must risk the possibility of being cited for contempt by Judge Scarlett and incarcerated. But one thing is certain: your profession owes you a tremendous debt of gratitude."

Bell was unquestionably one of the court's strongest civil rights enforcers while on the Fifth Circuit Court of Appeals, with jurisdiction over the Deep South states of Alabama, Florida, Georgia, Louisiana, Mississippi and Texas, which was the battleground in the struggle for civil rights. He was not, however, in favor of integration if it meant the forced busing of minorities to achieve a racial balance in every school. In Bell's opinion, forced busing fractured the fabric and strength of traditional neighborhoods.

Consequently, Carter's nomination of Bell as the nation's highest law enforcement officer created a firestorm of controversy and several liberal Democrats led the charge to derail his nomination. At best, Bell's civil rights record during his fourteen years on the Fifth Circuit bench was mixed and the New York Times and Wall Street Journal blasted Carter's decision. Reporters scoured every detail of Bell's personal life, turning up his memberships in two exclusive private clubs, the Capital City Club and the Piedmont Driving Club, infamous for barring blacks and Jews as members. Bell, to his credit, quit both clubs.

Realizing that my old friend's nomination was in jeopardy, I contacted Daddy King to discuss my feelings about the opposition and vituperative remarks. Dad was of the opinion that Griffin Bell was like most white Southern judges of his generation until I explained my experience with him during the Moore case as far back as 1968, a time when Bell was practically the only judge who supported my efforts. I told Dad that based upon my knowledge and experience with Griffin Bell that "he is not a racist. If he were, he had every opportunity to demonstrate it during the Moore case." Once convinced of Bell's character, Daddy King had no problem honoring my request to contact other prominent black leaders who were vehemently opposed to his nomination and asked them to tone down their verbal abuse.

Griffin Bell's confirmation hearing before the Senate Judiciary Committee was chaired by the arch conservative from Mississippi, Senator James Eastland. Several black leaders were still irate, in spite of Dad's intervention, and vowed to fight and block the nomination. At that point I called Senator Eastland's office and volunteered to appear before his committee and a staff member was assigned to interview me at great length, inquiring into my background and experience as well as Judge Bell's reputation.

The questions were blunt. "What do you know of Judge Bell's attitudes on race?" I was asked.

"I can tell you of my personal experience with him during my representation of an indigent black man accused of murdering two prominent white men in Southeast Georgia, back in 1966, and who was sentenced to death in the electric chair. He had every opportunity to demonstrate racial prejudice, and never at any time was that revealed.

And I would be pleased to appear before the Senate Judiciary Committee to testify on his behalf. Griffin Bell is not now, nor has he ever been a racist."

On January 10, 1977, I followed up my interview with Eastland's staff with a letter to the senator advising him that I would be pleased to appear before the committee to testify on behalf of Griffin Bell's nomination. One month to the day later I received a letter from Judge Bell: "I was given a copy of your letter to Senator Eastland and appreciate very much your support and offer to appear before the Senate Judiciary Committee on my behalf."

Bell's appointment was not the end of the matter. The firestorm of controversy continued unabated. It is my opinion that part of the debate was fuelled by the fact that Griffin Bell was a Southerner and a pal of Jimmy Carter's, among other "faults." Democratic factions who were still disappointed in Carter's victory over McGovern would not go quietly and set to work trying to derail the appointment. At this late hour I leaned on Daddy King to step up his efforts and one by one the objections of America's most prominent black leaders were withdrawn. After being subjected to one of the most contentious Senate confirmation fights in history, the Senate Judiciary Committee voted 10-3 to recommend Bell's confirmation. On January 25, the Senate voted 75-21 to confirm.

The new attorney general followed up his first letter to me with a second, dated February 17, in which he thanked me for my help in securing his appointment, and a third, on March 8, acknowledging my congratulatory note to him.

It is interesting to note that during his tenure as US Attorney General that Griffin Bell rebuilt the Justice Department as a neutral zone in government and restored the bruised and battered integrity of the Federal Bureau of Investigation after the Watergate fiasco. Needless to add, Bell was one of the most effective attorney generals in our nation's history, and upon his resignation in 1979, and his return to private practice in the Atlanta law firm of King & Spalding, the Chief Justice of the US Supreme Court Warren Burger said of Bell that "no finer man has ever occupied the great office of Attorney General of the United States or discharged his duties with greater distinction."

To that I say, "Well done, thou good and faithful servant!"

(Can I get an "amen" to that?" "AMEN")

Chapter Six

AMBASSADOR ANDY
AND THE
FATHER OF THE YEAR

Griffin Bell's appointment to Attorney General of the United States was not the only Carter selection to come under fire. In an open and direct effort to reward Daddy King for his outstanding contributions to the Carter campaign, the new president tapped Andy Young to be US Ambassador to the United Nations. Long before Carter's decision had been made public, Andy invited me to his office to weigh in on the subject, having canvassed his wife and Daddy King. As Andy's friend and counsel and campaign finance chairman I was in a unique position to outline the pros and cons of a black Baptist preacher becoming an international diplomat.

"Andy, I would not accept it," I said, flatly. "I think that with all you and Dad did for Jimmy Carter that he should give you a cabinet level appointment."

Andy looked at me in amazement. "Really? I'm surprised, I really am, because you're the only one who feels that way. Jean is in favor..."

"You asked me for my opinion and you're not paying me for it. I'm speaking from the heart, what I think is best for you."

"Well, I must say you certainly speak your mind. You don't bite your tongue." I think Andy was actually looking for something more along the lines of "congratulations."

"Look, Andy, I know you. And I know that you are not going to be happy stuck away from the action. The UN isn't where the action is. There is no political future after the UN. Diplomacy can be a lifetime job, but it's a dead end job. Besides, you have some very strong opinions about matters that may cause you problems. Israel, for example..."

Andy looked at me straight in the eye. "Thank you, Murray. I appreciate your opinion, but I'm going to accept the president's offer."

We shook hands and parted company.

A few weeks later, Barbara and I attended Andy's swearing in ceremony in the Gold Room of the White House. We sat directly in front of Hubert Humphrey.

Controversial from the start, Andy was baptized by fire for his remarks regarding efforts to normalize relations with Nigeria, which had been torn apart by civil war, assassinations and corruption, for his stand on ending segregation in Zimbabwe Rhodesia, and for his position that Cuban troops brought stability to Angola. Then in 1979, Andy met with members of the Palestinian Liberation Organization (PLO), contrary to and in direct intervention with federal policy and law. The original charter of the PLO spelled out its goal of liberating the homeland from Israel by any means necessary, and went so far as to declare the nation of Israel "illegal, null and void." When Andy's secret meetings with the PLO leadership was revealed, he tried to duck and cover, which the media perceived as evasive. Publicity mounted, pressure from the Jewish community increased and it all began to take a toll on Andy's health. He became paranoid and feared that his telephone lines were tapped by the FBI. He sent word through Bennette that he wanted to meet with me at my earliest convenience at his office in Atlanta, under the guise of returning home to visit his family and Coretta.

We met the following day. Andy wasted no time in coming to the point of the matter:

"Murray, you've been following this situation with the PLO?"

"Yes, sir..."

"Well, what do you think? Will it blow over? Seriously, what do you think?"

"I think this is a mess," I said, picking up where we had left off in the prior conversation about his appointment. "You will recall that I counseled you not to accept this appointment, that Israel might be a problem for you. No doubt in my mind the Jews will raise hell about this, and you're gonna put Jimmy Carter between a rock and a hard place. He's gonna fire you, that is if you don't resign. He'll have no choice."

"That bad, huh? You really feel that way?"

"I really do," I said, and it gave me no pleasure to say so.

"I have one or two others I need to talk to," Andy concluded. "I'll let you know." And with that, there was nothing left to say. A few days later I got a call from Bennette, advising me of Andy's decision to resign.

Andy Young was indeed fortunate to have had two brilliant parents. In September 1977, they came to visit their sons in Atlanta, and Jean Young invited Barbara and me to meet them. Andrew Young, Sr. was a dentist in New Orleans; his wife Daisy was a teacher. We had met on three prior occasions, the first being when we took them to dinner at our favorite restaurant, the second, when Andy was sworn in as Ambassador to the United Nations. The third was a surprise, when I met then in New York, on my first visit to the Ambassador's new office, and we were given the VIP tour of the UN. I keep a lovely note I received from Daisy Young, dated September 28, 1977, in which she thanks me for a lovely evening, saying, "It was good to know you and I feel that I had known you for many years." Then the meeting in Washington was an added pleasure." The letter goes on to include an invitation for Barbara and me to visit the Youngs in their home and to meet a friend who was running for mayor of New Orleans.

It was plain to see that the apple does not fall far from the tree. Andy's parents were activists and took an interest in their local politics and on a national scale; articulate, serious, friendly.

I also recall around this time that Daddy King was admitting to feeling rather poorly, as he put it, and lacking energy, which was code for an empty pantry. Steak was his favorite remedy, but plagued with dental discomfort, the meat had to be extra tender. I ordered a dozen of the finest AAA prime steaks from an exclusive company in Colorado, and specified that each was to be cut one inch and a half thick and drop shipped overnight to Dad's residence. He received the package and called me promptly to say, "Counsel, you shouldn't have done this. It will take me three months to eat all these steaks."

"Dad, do your best," I replied. "I got faith in you."

When I called him back eight days later, his housekeeper answered the call.

"How are those steaks holding out?" I asked her.

"Sir, they're all gone but two. Reverend Bennette took two, Marty took two, and Dad sent some to Mrs. Coretta."

He was too good; he was priceless.

I think of Daddy King and I am reminded of John Wesley's quote:

> *"Do all the good you can,*
> *By all the means you can,*
> *In all the ways you can,*
> *In all the places you can,*
> *To all the people you can,*
> *As long as you can."*

Here endeth the lesson.

All things considered, 1977 was a pretty good year for Daddy King. He was front and center on the day that President Carter awarded the Presidential Medal of Freedom to Martin Luther King, Jr. posthumously, the highest civilian award in the United States. Established in 1945 by President Truman, the award is given annually to recipients selected by the president and is designed to honor those individuals who have made "an especially meritorious contribution to the security or national interests of the

United States, world peace, cultural or other significant public or private endeavors." Other activists so honored include Andrew Young, Jr., Rosa Parks, James Farmer, and Whitney M. Young, Jr.

In presenting the award, President Carter said that Martin Luther King, Jr. was the "conscience of his generation." In accepting the award on behalf of her husband, Coretta Scott King announced that it would be placed on permanent display in the King Center.

"His Excellency Andrew Young, Chairman, the Vice Chairpersons, the Committee and Mrs. Coretta Scott King, President, request the honor of your presence at the First Annual Dinner of the Martin Luther King, Jr. Center for Non-Violent Social Change honoring the Reverend Doctor Martin Luther King, Sr. Wednesday, October 12, 1977—New York Hilton—Grand Ballroom—RSVP—Dress Optional—Reception 6 o'clock, Dinner 7 o'clock."

Barbara and I attended, in formal attire, and were greeted at the entrance by Rev. Bennette, who was also formally dressed, much to his satisfaction and pleasure.

On December 19, we were invited to Daddy King's 78th birthday party, a gathering of family and close friends at Coretta's residence. The party was in full swing by 7:30 when the telephone rang and Christine King Farris answered the phone. "There's a call for you, Dad, from the president," she said, handing her father the receiver.

Answering, "Yes, President Carter," he heard the president say, "I want you to know just how much I appreciate your support and friendship without which I could not have been elected president."

Affirmation of fact by the man himself.

It was a sentiment oft repeated while Jimmy Carter was in office. At the Black Leaders Convention held in Atlanta on September 16, 1980, Mayor Maynard Jackson presiding, with Daddy King and Coretta in attendance, Carter told attendees, "If it hadn't been for Daddy King and his beloved wife, I would not be president."

(EDITORIAL NOTE: *As recently as February 7, 2006, in an interview with Wolf Blitzer on the CNN news program* The Situation Room, *Jimmy Carter acknowledged, "When Coretta and Daddy King adopted me in 1976, it legitimized a southern governor as an acceptable candidate for president. Each of their public handshakes to me was worth a million Yankee votes."*)

In May 1978, Rev. Bennette (who had vowed never to fly again after retrieving ML's body from Memphis) asked me to accompany Dad to New York City for "The National Father of the Year Award," presented annually since 1931 by business leaders and concerned citizens forming the Fathers Day Council, to achieve universal observance of the little known holiday. The purpose of the award was to confer honors upon contemporary leaders of our society, and the list of recipients includes Arthur Ashe, Ossie Davis, George Will, General Norman Schwarzkopf, Colin Powell, and eighty others.

Bennette drove Daddy King and me to the airport. We flew first class front row, and were met at the plane by a chauffeur driven black Cadillac limousine. We arrived in time for the luncheon and were seated at the head table with other recipients: actor Yul Brynner, Speaker of the

House Tip O'Neil, columnist William Safire, and, last but not least, one of my personal heroes, "The Yankee Captain," Thurman Munson.

O'Neil greeted us warmly and hugged Dad, and then introduced us to the other honorees. Since the founding of the award in 1931, the National Fathers Day Committee had selected only two "Religious Father of the Year," the first being Rev. Billy Graham, in 1957, and Daddy King, in 1978. Not too shabby for a poor country boy from Georgia.

It was indeed gratifying to watch the genuine outpouring of respect and admiration for Rev. King, by far, the biggest man in attendance.

Our return trip that same afternoon was most pleasant. Bennette was waiting for us at the Atlanta airport and drove us to our respective homes. En route Bennette asked Dad, "Did my lawyer take good care of you?" to which Dad replied, "Yes, Bennette. I cannot complain, he recognized *everybody.*"

Life gives us a handful of brief moments with others, but sometimes, in those brief moments, we form memories that last a lifetime.

(EDITORIAL NOTE, and a tragic one, at that: *Thurman Munson, the New York Yankee catcher since 1969, had collected a string of accolades, including Rookie of the Year, American League All-Star, MVP, and the only other player since the great Lou Gehrig to be elected team captain by his teammates, was killed in a private airplane crash on August 2, 1979. A Fathers Day does not pass without my remembering Munson and Daddy King.*)

Chapter Seven

A Theory
Goes On Trial

At the end of July 1980, an article published by the *Atlanta Constitution* receiving little notice drastically changed my professional life and created the greatest dilemma of my career. The reporter of the story, Roger Witherspoon, contributed a piece on the subject of race, intelligence and eugenics (the study of hereditary improvement of the human race by controlled selective breeding), and linked recent efforts by a Nobel laureate in Physics to point up the problem of the black population down breeding lower intelligence to Adolf Hitler's creation of a master race. Witherspoon, who happened to be of African-American ancestry, took offense with the position held by William B. Shockley that the higher rate of reproduction among the less intelligent was having a dysgenic effect, and that a drop in average intelligence would ultimately lead to a decline in civilization. Shockley not only advocated that the scientific community should investigate heredity, intelligence and demographic trends, he went further in suggesting that there should be corrective governmental policy changes should he be proven right, and it was his ultimate solution that individuals with IQs below 100 be paid to undergo voluntary sterilization. As Witherspoon pointed out, such policies would effectively wipe out the Negro race, and in voicing his disapproval of the plan and the notions behind it, the writer went so far as to refer to the 70-year-old founder of Silicon Valley as a "Hitlerite," which earned the disapproval of Dr. Shockley.

Dr. Shockley filed suit. Being a resident of California, he needed legal representation in Georgia, and was directed to the eminent counsel, Hon. Judge J. Walter Cowart of Savannah, who demanded a retraction from the newspaper which was denied. Whereupon Judge Cowart filed suit for Libel on behalf of Shockley in the US District Court, Northern District of Georgia, Atlanta Division, in the sum of $1,250,000, against AJC publisher Cox Enterprises, Inc. Being a public figure, the burden of proof that his reputation had been damaged by Witherspoon's article was on Dr. Shockley, and in order to prevail Judge Cowart was going to have to prove that not only was Witherspoon wrong, he was also guilty of actual malice in publishing his attack.

The reputation that writer Witherspoon had sullied was considerable, beginning all the way back in 1938, when the recent honor grad from MIT received his first patent for an electron multiplier. An employee of the famous Bell Labs in New Jersey, he headed up a new division of radar research during World War II, devising methods for countering submarine tactics and the advent of new radar bomb sights. For this project, Secretary of War Robert Patterson awarded Shockley the Medal of Merit in 1946. But it was the quiet calculations of this unknown physicist that forever changed the world: in July 1945, the War Department asked Shockley to prepare a report on the probable casualties resulting from an invasion of the Japanese mainland in which he surmised that in order for the US to succeed American forces would have to kill at least 5 to 10 million Japanese at a cost between 1.7 and 4 million allied casualties, and it was these calculations that convinced the top brass that the atomic bombings of Hiroshima and Nagasaki was the best way to achieve the goal without making the sacrifice.

After the war, Bell Labs returned to more peaceful pursuits and Dr. Shockley headed up the team assigned with finding a solid-state alternative to the fragile glass vacuum tube amplifier, based on Shockley's ideas about using an external electrical field on a semiconductor to affect its conductivity. By 1947, Shockley's team had come up with the world's first point-contact transistor. A falling out between team members over ownership of patents caused him to break rank and set off on his solo quest to refine the semiconductor, resulting in the publication of the book that became the bible for an entire generation of scientists working to develop and improve the transistor. By 1951, Shockley had improved upon the point-contact transistor with his new junction transistor, which became the application of choice in the marketplace. For his accomplishments, Shockley was elected a member of the National Academy of Sciences (NAS), who then conferred upon him the prestigious Comstock Prize for Physics, a spate of awards and honors to follow.

He did not play well with other inventors. The ensuing publicity Shockley received as "Father of the Transistor" pissed off the other members of his Bell Labs team that had worked on the project in its incubating stage to the point that he blocked them from working on his junction transistor. Shockley wanted the power and profit he felt he deserved and his abrasive management style caused him to be passed over for executive promotion. He left Bell Labs in 1953, returned to Caltech, where he had earned his BS, and linked up with Beckman Instruments to develop the "Shockley Diode" (now known as the thyristor).

Shockley was a co-recipient of the Nobel Prize in Physics in 1956, along with the team members with whom he had differed, and the sharing of the world's most prestigious honor healed the rift between them.

And then an odd thing happened to the good doctor that forever changed the face of technology and his personal fortunes: eight of his researchers resigned in 1957, after Shockley decided to abandon research into the silicon-based semiconductor, several of whom then started up Fairchild Semiconductor. Among the "traitors" were Robert Noyce and Gordon Moore, the future founders of Intel and its offspring National Semiconductor and Advanced Micro Devices. While Shockley was still piddling with a three-state device, Fairchild and Texas Instruments introduced the first integrated circuits, which effectively rendered the "Father of the Transistor" obsolete.

A near-fatal automobile accident in 1961 sidelined Dr. Shockley for several months during which his firm was sold off. He then joined Stanford University, where he taught Engineering and Applied Science. His last patent was granted in 1968, for a rather complex semiconductor, and when next the world heard of William Shockley he had reemerged as some sort of self-appointed expert in solving human problems through scientific ingenuity with an emphasis on genetics.

Although his first findings appeared to be more concerned with a drop in average intelligence throughout society, he found the situation among blacks to be disastrous and his position was quickly deemed political, not scientific. Shockley published findings that showed unskilled whites had 3.7 children on average versus an average of 2.3 children for skilled whites, but that unskilled blacks had 5.4 children versus 1.9 for skilled blacks. At that rate, Shockley reasoned, intelligence, which like most traits is inherited, would decline and that at some point American inner cities would be populated by big and strong but ignorant black people and that the government would not be able to build jails fast enough to deal with the resulting crime. Considering the options, Shockley deemed it advisable that the government pay individuals with IQs below 100 to undergo voluntary sterilization, which was designed not only to reduce the fastest growing segment of the most inferior segment of society but to alleviate the inability of the welfare system to meet the growing demand as well as the penal system.

Shockley's views made sense on paper to many observers, but none of them were black. All Roger Witherspoon could read into Shockley's findings was that whites were genetically superior to blacks and the fear of what the world might look like in one hundred years should growth among the unskilled continue unabated somehow entitled the government to adopt a solution similar to the Nazi view of cleansing the racially impure. Roger Witherspoon wasn't in favor of genocide and he said so in his article denouncing Dr. Shockley.

Walter Cowart spent months pressing Shockley's case through litigation and discovery during which he attracted a measure of attention and publicity, most of it hostile to Shockley. At one point he was waylaid by a reporter who asked him bluntly, "Isn't it true that this suit is all about money?" to which Shockley replied, "No, it is not all about money. If I recover one dollar I will be satisfied; it is about my reputation." Words he would come to regret when settlement rolled around.

The stress of the Shockley case was more than Judge Cowart could handle, his heart giving out long before the process was over. Acting on doctor's orders, Cowart advised Shockley that he had gone as far as his ailing heart could take him and could go no further. In suggesting his able replacement, Cowart said to Shockley, "I have known Murray Silver for over twenty-five years. He is honest, hard working, capable, experienced, and maybe the best trial lawyer in the state of Georgia, with the guts and determination to provide outstanding learned counsel,"— or, at least that's what Dr. Shockley said Cowart told him in his initial conversation with me two days later.

During my initial review of the Shockley case it seemed a shame that the accomplishments of this great scientist should be misinterpreted as racist and demonized by the popular media who created an unbalanced picture of his beliefs and opinions. Nowhere had he set out to launch political doctrines in the name of eugenics which could be used to exterminate a race, but in setting out to scientifically explore the influences that improve inborn qualities his purpose became easily misunderstood by those who misused his findings to further their own agendas—and by those who were forced to defend its perceived target by any means necessary.

After reviewing the case files that had been amassed by Judge Cowart (who ably assisted me throughout the trial, along with my son Eric), I had a remarkable initial consultation with Dr. Shockley to find out from him exactly what was behind his decision to file a suit for libel, what were his intentions, and what was his desired outcome. He appeared in my office looking very much like the quintessential college professor: small of stature, balding grey hair, bespectacled piercing eyes, a well-worn tweed jacket, he had the appearance of a Muppet had Jim Henson created a Professor character. He somehow established a likeable balance between being one of the most brilliant minds of the twentieth century and his college's most popular professor through a cunning sense of humor (providing you were quick enough and smart enough to understand his references), his interest in magic and a reputation as a prankster. I found him to be pleasant company and nothing like the "Hitlerite" he had been painted in Roger Witherspoon's portrait.

For Dr. Shockley, his case was centered on Witherspoon's comment that there was nothing new about Shockley's findings and that the "Shockley program was tried out in Germany during World War II, when scientists under direction of the government experimented on Jews and defectives in an effort to study genetic development," and went even further in asserting that "for Shockley the German experiments weren't wrong per se." Those statements, in Dr. Shockley's opinion, were wrong in that his interest in eugenics developed many years after the war was over, that he had not provided Nazi Germany with a program of any kind, and false in the assertion that Shockley agreed with the experiments conducted in the concentration camps. Not only were these comments wrong and false, it was Dr. Shockley's contention that the writer Witherspoon knew that they were defective as such and designed to subject him to ridicule, contempt and public hatred, thereby lessening his worth as a scientist and humanitarian, warping the value placed on his accomplishments, forever negatively impacting the future of his recorded history, and denigrating his reputation as a productive and useful citizen. The spirit of the entire article was malicious; filled with false statements, half-truths and sly innuendo. In presenting Shockley as the architect of the Holocaust—or at a minimum that he approved of those horrible experiments—was to falsely charge him with crimes against humanity, and that was something the good doctor would not allow to stand.

Litigation in federal courts can be an almost endless process. After Judge Cowart handed off the Shockley case to me in July 1982, a number of heretofore unknown events transpired that have a direct bearing on the spirit and purpose of this book.

As soon as I filed my appearance in the matter as attorney of record, I was deluged with telephone calls, some complimentary and congratulatory, others inquisitive and concerned. My good friend Kirk McAlpin, former president of the American Bar Association, called to say "great news for the old Savannah boy." I received a similar slap on the back from the Hon. H. Sol Clark, Judge, Georgia Court of Appeals, and Hon. Charles Weltner, Chief Justice, Georgia Supreme Court. Andrew Young was more reserved in his enthusiasm when he called to inquire, "Why you?" My response: "Why not me? I am well qualified, and frankly speaking, with the racial overtones, perhaps no one else is better suited." Andy paused, and in that pause I have thought back over these events and wondered what he might've thought but was too polite to say, and abruptly ended the conversation, saying, "Well, I hope it all works out."

Quite frankly, I expected an extreme reaction from certain corners, but the reader should be advised that before consenting to represent Dr. Shockley I discussed the ramifications at length with my family, to whom I owed my highest consideration, especially since both of my sons had followed me into law school and both were in my employ, and then sought the sage counsel of Daddy King. The very last thing I was prepared to sacrifice was my relationship with him and Coretta and the King family, and so I paid Dad a call and laid out the entire matter.

Of all the conversations I ever had with the thousands of clients that I represented during a career that spanned almost 45 years, none can compare with the complexities both mental and emotional involved in explaining to Rev. Martin Luther King, Sr. why I wanted to come to the aid and assistance of Dr. William Shockley at a time when no other lawyer in the State of Georgia wanted the case; it was Robert Felton Moore all over again—but in racial reverse. I drew a very deep breath and chose my words with extraordinary care as I explained to Dad that Dr. Shockley was the first scientist to break the taboo on frank discussion of racial differences and that his research delved into the intricacies of how intelligence is linked to race, leading to his recommendation that the government take certain actions to prevent the lower end of the spectrum from becoming the most dominant. I explained that a black writer had been so disturbed by Shockley's findings that he had been prompted to write an article attacking him as a racist and worse, and without pausing to take a second deep breath told Dad that the most important thing I wanted him to know was that this was a libel suit, not a forum for genetic or racial theories, and that it was my intention to "stay close to the book" and prevent the trial from becoming a circus.

And then the Rev. King said something that took me by complete surprise: rather than launch into an attack of his own, or a defense of his race, or a statement as to his feelings, he said to me, "Counsel, how does all this make you feel?"

It was not a question that anyone else had bothered to consider and I felt a lump rise in my throat at the recognition of his remarkable compassion for my plight, as only Daddy King could have. "How do you *feel*?" he repeated, stressing the last word.

At that moment I felt a strong urge to cry merely out of the frustration I felt for causing Dad to worry about me. I have always thought that if someone was worried about me that it meant I wasn't doing a very good job, and I did not want Dad to worry about me. "Dad, I am not the lawyer that filed the original suit; this was not my idea. I inherited this case from an old friend who couldn't withstand the physical stress; this case put him in the hospital. I want you to know that while I do not agree with my client's theories, he—as a Nobel laureate—has a right to his opinion and I will forever defend his right to free speech. I want you to know first and foremost that this is a libel case, that the newspaper goes too far in labeling him a Nazi, and that it is the newspaper that introduced race into the matter, not Dr. Shockley. Dr. Shockley did not launch some sort of attack on black people that Mr. Witherspoon was forced to defend. Mr. Witherspoon attacked Dr. Shockley as the architect of the Holocaust, which is outrageous. If anyone should feel any animosity toward Dr. Shockley it should be the Jews—if what Witherspoon says about him is true—and I know I need not remind you that I am Jewish. If I thought for a single second that Shockley was a racist or a Nazi, we would not be having this discussion..."

Dad rocked back and studied me intently.

"If nothing else, Dr. Shockley is entitled to a fair hearing and the best legal counsel available," I said, in conclusion. "In Judge Cowart's opinion, that counsel is me."

"Counsel," Dad said, his voice rising as if delivering an invocation, "I understand and I agree that Dr. Shockley could not do better than you. Counsel wisely," he said, patting my hand. "I appreciate your coming here today and telling me what I know had to be difficult for you to say. We're together. Thank you."

And in that moment of grace and benediction, the father of the civil rights movement enabled me to take up the cause of America's first "scientific racist." Thereafter, when other black acquaintances chastised me for what they felt was an ill-considered decision, my patent response was, "Daddy King doesn't have a problem with it. What's yours?"

I maintain in my personal files a stack of letters and telegrams collected through the years, many of which were received during the Shockley years, including one from the

Imperial Wizard of the Knights of the Ku Klux Klan, bearing a Mississippi postmark, advising me that I would be hearing from them soon on a matter of "national emergency." One week later I received a follow-up telephone call advising me that a group of Klansmen would be calling on me to discuss matters of extreme importance and please permit them the opportunity to be heard. Three hours later, a trio arrived at my office and advised me that they wanted to form an exploratory committee in support of Shockley running for president of the United States. Their reason for coming to me was to entice me with $50,000 to get my client to go along with the plan. As was my obligation to my client, I advised the Klansmen that I would take up the matter with Dr. Shockley and that I would have a response within a week. "You know," one of the Klansmen said, as they were exiting the office, "if it would help you in his trial we could organize a parade down Peachtree Street." I thanked him for his generosity but declined, saying that the trial was difficult enough without any demonstrations or further distractions.

Oddly, Dr. Shockley was flattered by the Klan's interest. I really didn't think that he would pay the notion any mind, reminding him that any affiliation with the Ku Klux Klan at this particular point in the litigation of his case would not be in his best interests. The matter was rejected and dropped, much to the disappointment of the boys from Mississippi.

The Shockley case garnered a tremendous amount of international publicity; interviews alone took up an incredible amount of time. Letters, telegrams, phone calls, reporters, newspapers, magazines, television—you name it, we got it. Many attempts both blatant and veiled sought to make the case into a litmus test of Shockley's controversial theories on race. It was my contention then—as it is now—that it was never about race; this is a libel suit, that's all. The *Atlanta Journal-Constitution*, as the bully pulpit, tried to bully prospective jurors by publishing a spate of stories that shaded the issues at stake. Other newspapers picked up the *AJC* cue: *Miami Herald, New York Times, Boston Globe, Los Angeles Times, London Times, Newsweek, Time, US News and World Report. American Jurisprudence* cited Shockley as one of the ten most important cases of 1984.

But because I did not want the case tried in the media I instructed Dr. Shockley to refrain from any and all interviews. Difficult at first, due to his desire to make himself understood, he would talk at length anytime a microphone was shoved in his face. He soon discovered that no matter what he said, his statements were twisted by the commentary made before and after and he learned the hard way to distrust a media hell-bent on coming to the assistance of their brother writer defendant. Shockley attempted to hold the media more accountable by taping interviews with reporters and then sending a transcript to the reporter by registered mail. He even resorted to making reporters take a quiz on his work before discussing anything of consequence with them. I had a greater concern, however, that his famous statement to a reporter at the onset of the process would come back to haunt him: "If I recover one dollar I will be satisfied; it is about my reputation." I did not want the case tried in the media; I wanted the case tried in court.

I got my wish. The newspaper refused to settle, and jury selection began and was completed, on September 5,

1984: six jurors, one black.

I had a stellar line up of witnesses for the plaintiff, including Clark Mollenhoff, the Pulitzer Prize winning syndicated columnist, Washington correspondent, lawyer, and author of ten books. Mollenhoff was the well-known Deputy Counsel to President Nixon, and Special Counsel, 1969-70, and will forever be remembered as the insider whose sad task it was to inform Nixon that he had no other alternative but to resign the presidency, saying, "It's time to go, Mr. President." My purpose for introducing Mollenhoff was to have him hold forth on The Code of Ethics of the Society of Professional Journalists and The Basic Statement of Principles of the National Conference of Editorial Writers. Any witness the defense intended to produce that planned to testify as to opinions based on false statements would clearly be at odds with Mollenhoff, a most imposing figure and one helluva witness. He not only spoke with a professorial authority, he delivered his teachings in a voice that shook the courthouse rafters. And quickly, word spread throughout the courthouse and the Atlanta legal community at large that the best free show in town was being played out in Judge Vining's courtroom.

In addition to Clark Mollenhoff, I presented Prof. Richard Hernstein from Harvard; Dr. Leonard Heston from the University of Minnesota; Prof. AR Jensen from the University of California Berkeley; and Prof. Arthur Steinberg from Case Western as witnesses for Shockley, all of whom roundly denounced Witherspoon's unwarranted attack with pen and ink. Having laid a solid foundation of ethics and responsibilities from the nation's leading teachers on the subject of Journalism, I produced the man himself to testify in a verbal volley that lasted ninety minutes, highlighted with his impassioned claim that Witherspoon's accusation that the "Shockley Program" was tried out in Germany during World War II was a "damnable, evil lie." It was a most decisive point and the force with which it was served made quite an impression on the jury and spectators that jammed every bench in the courtroom. And then, upon cross examination by the newspaper's attorneys, all the good I had done the good doctor came undone when he repeated the famous "One Dollar" quote, and it was still fresh in the jury's mind when they set about their deliberations.

Perhaps *Time* magazine summed it up best:

"Murray Silver, Shockley's fire breathing Atlanta lawyer, acknowledged his own disagreement with his client's theories but insisted that Shockley's views were irrelevant to the case. He charged the defense with trying to divert attention from the essential point, that the Constitution printed Witherspoon's contention with malice. "They knew it was false when they published it." Silver used witnesses like Pulitzer Prize winning reporter Clark Mollenhoff, now a Professor of Journalism and Law at Washington and Lee University, who called the article "...a whole mishmash of false information."

"Silver also singled out a 1979 Constitution column in which Witherspoon falsely claimed that a cerebral palsy victim named Arnold participated in an Atlanta running competition. "I wrote it that way to prove a point," was Witherspoon's somewhat weak defense on the stand. "I assumed everybody knew he wasn't there." Hammering away at the reporter's reliability, Silver told the courtroom, "Accusations of criminal activity, even in the form of expressions of opinion, are not constitutionally protected."

Witherspoon, he said, had charged Shockley with crimes against humanity.

"After just three and a halfhours of deliberation, the six-member jury—five whites and one black—returned with a remarkable evenhanded decision. The Verdict: Shockley had been libeled. The damage to his reputation: $1.00. Said Shockley, who had asked for a "conspicuous" penalty: "This will encourage the press to take equal freedom in libeling others."

(*Time*, Sept. 24, 1984, page 62, "A Theory Goes on Trial," by Richard Lacayo, Reported by B. Russell Leavitt/ Atlanta).

(EDITORIAL NOTE: *In 1999,* Time *magazine published "Time 100: The 100 Great Minds of the Century," which, along with Albert Einstein, Sigmund Freud and the Wright Brothers, prominently listed Dr. William B. Shockley.*)

Chapter Eight

The Least
Of These

It wasn't often that Rev. Bennette called me about a security-related problem at the King Center, but I distinctly remember the events of Friday, June 15, 1979, when he asked me to meet him at the site on Auburn Avenue; I was there in fifteen minutes. I found Bennette in an agitated state with a pudgy, young black man who had been loitering around the property with a camera, intent on interviewing Mrs. King. When Bennette asked the man for some sort of identification, the man refused, saying he was a "news photographer." Bennette attempted to search the man's case—as was his custom as the Center's chief of security—but the man refused to cooperate and it was at this point that Bennette ordered him off the premises. The man refused to leave, and Bennette called me rather than involve the police. I arrived on the scene to find Bennette engaged in a bizarre argument with the man:

"...I can wait here as long as I want to and you can't stop me," I overheard the man shout at Bennette.

"If you come back here again, I will have you arrested for trespass," Bennette countered. "Here's my attorney now..."

"What's the problem here?" I asked the man. "I'm Murray Silver, a member of the board here and Mrs. King's counsel. May I ask who you are, sir?

"My name is Wayne Williams. I live in Dixie Hills, and the rest is none of your damn business!" With that, he turned and walked away, not to be seen or heard from again, at least, not until two years later when I got a call from Dr. Bernard Bridges, asking me if I had any interest in defending a young black man being held as a key suspect in the Atlanta Child Murders, occurring between 1979 and 1981.

"I've met the man," I told Dr. Bridges, "and I'm fairly certain that he wouldn't want me to represent him, owing to the nature of our initial introduction."

Hardly two weeks passed before I got a call from Daddy King, asking me why Atlanta's best criminal lawyer wasn't representing Atlanta's worst criminal. I related the strange tale of Rev. Bennette encountering Wayne Williams at the Center, confirmed by Bennette. Wayne, who had been arrested on June 21, 1981, for the murder of two young black men, stood trial in January 1982, and was found guilty after deciding to take the stand in his own defense and was a hostile witness, to say the least. I was contacted by Wayne's attorneys and requested to handle the appeal, which I declined.

The Wayne Williams murder case reminded me of the first time I met Rev. Bennette during the Robert Felton Moore trial in Camden County, Georgia, in 1966. He had accompanied Martin Luther King, Jr. to the site to find out for themselves how the trial was proceeding and whether the defendant was being treated fairly. Fearing that Moore was going to be lynched by an angry mob, they were surprised to find a white lawyer beating back the tides of racial hate and prejudice instead. Out of this auspicious meeting began a great friendship that lasted nearly thirty years.

Born in Atlanta and reared in the Buttermilk Bottom section of the city, Bennette had joined the army straight out of graduating from Howard High, attained the rank of Sergeant, and at the end of his hitch entered into the Turner Theological Seminary at Morris Brown College, where he was introduced to the King brothers, Martin and AD, in 1960. He was a proud member of Ebenezer Baptist Church and became a key organizer in the Southern Christian Leadership Conference (SCLC) that same year. One of Bennette's first projects was targeting Atlanta's landmark business, Rich's Department Store, by staging a sit-in for desegregation. The success of the Rich's campaign elevated Bennette to Director of Voter Registration and Deputy Director of the Georgia Voters League. In 1964, Martin appointed him the first director of SCLC's "Operation Bread Basket," a feed-the-hungry initiative, where he served with distinction for three years. All the while Rev. Bennette was Pastor of Mount Welcome Baptist Church, located in Atlanta's Pittsburg community.

Had it not been necessary for Bennette to undergo a tracheotomy to relieve a blockage in the windpipe, resulting in his voice being hampered by a deep hoarseness and laborious breathing, he would without a doubt have been an outstanding leader on the order of Hosea Williams and

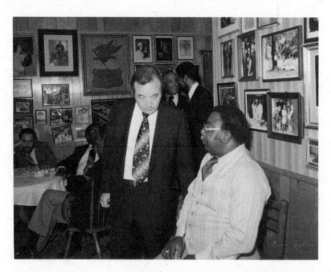

Fred Bennette and Silver in the King residence.

Ralph Abernathy. As such, Bennette was behind the scenes, and it is a little known fact that he advised Jimmy Carter on issues of importance to the black community during Carter's bid for the governorship of Georgia. In fact, it was Bennette who arranged for Carter to meet Daddy King. But it was his undying dedication to Andrew Young that Bennette is best remembered, working 24/7 in Andy's bids for Congress, for Mayor of Atlanta, and for Governor of Georgia. Bennette was on Andy's staff until the day he died in 1994.

The biographical note about Bennette that I want to illuminate is a little known but rather important event that happened during a rally for the Freedom Riders in Montgomery, Alabama, in 1961. At the time, Bennette was an SCLC organizer, planning protests and organizing marches in Martin's Southern campaign for civil rights. A bomb was thrown at Martin that landed at his feet. Acting without hesitation, Bennette picked it up and tossed it away, out of harm's way. Rarely is this remarkable act of sacrifice and courage mentioned in the annals of civil rights history.

I often kidded my dear friend that he was miserable if he did not know every second the whereabouts of Andy Young and every member of the King family. Bennette was incredibly protective of them all and dedicated his life to their safety and well being. He had a black book like no other, filled with reams of telephone numbers of people across the country, whom he never hesitated to call on any matter, at any time, any place. Knowledge is power, and the best way for anybody to find out anything was to contact Bennette.

My dear friend often kidded me in return, that in all the years we had been friends I had never so much as invited him to my house for dinner. After such an aside, I saw that what began in jest had become a more serious suggestion, and at long last invited him to join us for Sunday dinner in the summer of 1978. Barbara prepared a standing rib roast and carted out the crystal and fine china, the silverware and cloth napkins. We spent a pleasant afternoon talking as friends do; Bennette was no stranger to my family. During the course of dinner Bennette took my sons to school on what it was like to be in service to Martin Luther King back in the day, when they had gone to Chicago and moved into a slum on the city's west side in order to dramatize the plight of public housing and urban decay. He recalled those hard, tough, cold days in the North Lawndale apartment in a three-flight walk-up, which they rented for $90 a month, but with their notoriety the landlord was shamed into improving the building quickly. Bennette went on to describe the Chicago operation, wherein he organized protests, tenant unions, marches, rallies, and rent strikes, until open housing finally became a reality. It was a lovely afternoon, at the end of which Bennette said as I walked him to his car, "I'm gonna call Jimmy Carter tomorrow and tell him I had dinner at your house!"

I thought that this too, was one of his jokes on me, but Bennette was earnest. The next day he called Jimmy Carter to say, "I had dinner at Murray Silver's house yesterday and his house is bigger than yours!" And that became one of his favorite jokes to tell on Carter in days to come.

Rev. Fred Bennette did not have much money. Many was the Sunday that he passed around the collection plate and got nothing in the way of folding money. If he was down to his last five dollars and he encountered someone with less, he wouldn't think twice of handing it over. I will never forget the day when we were having lunch at his favorite fried fish joint and he asked me for a little "sugar," as he was in need. I gave him twenty dollars. Lunch completed, I drove him home and as we passed an elderly black woman standing on the corner of Auburn Avenue, with what looked like all of her earthly possessions packed into plastic shopping bags, Bennette shouted, "Stop the car!" He got out of my car and approached the woman and gave her the twenty dollars. When he returned, he said, "Inasmuch you have done it unto one of the least of these, you have done it unto me," and the rest of the trip was spent in silence.

I do not believe that from the moment we moved to Atlanta in 1967 and meeting Fred Bennette that hardly a week went by without our having talked. I am eternally grateful that he arranged for me to meet Daddy King.

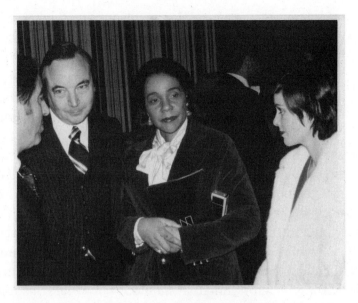

RCA Records reception for "Keep the Dream Alive Album," 1976

On several occasions Coretta Scott King and I shared the speaker's podium at various organizations and clubs, and regardless of the time or place Bennette was always present in his role as chief of security. He never missed an event but always missed the party, preferring to stand guard out front to protect Coretta from an enemy that never came. Bennette might even show up at a formal event in evening attire—nobody was more resplendent—but spend the entire affair on guard at or near the entrance; he was that protective of his friends. (Some of my favorite photos with Bennette are at some of these affairs and can be found throughout this book.) Years later, when Andy Young was Mayor of Atlanta and appointed me to a municipal judgeship, Rev. Bennette instructed his counterpart at the court house to "take care of Judge Silver," and thereafter I never left the building at the end of the day that an officer did not accompany me to my vehicle.

When the occasion called for formal attire, Bennette would always accompany me to Mitchell's Tuxedo, for he knew I would not make a big ceremony about picking up his tab, and I tell this minor fact to the reader for this reason: I am reminded of a time in March 1984, when Bennette casually mentioned to me that Dad needed a new suit. It was approaching Easter, and Bennette remarked that Dad had said something about wanting a white silk suit that he could wear to church on the high holiday. "You wouldn't happen to know where Dad could find a white silk suit, do you?" Bennette asked me, which was his subtle hint that should I know where this suit could be found that it would become a gift from me to Dad. Daddy King was a big man, and this suit wasn't going to be found on the rack at any men's shop; this suit was going to have to be tailored, and its price was beyond Dad's budget.

To make a gift of a tailored suit is to require making the offer to the recipient in such a way as not to embarrass, but to honor, and I saw the opportunity the next time I took Dad and Bennette to lunch. Max Epstein, who had run a tailor shop across the street from the court house for fifty years, was notified in advance of our arrival. Bruce Tielhaber, affable owner of Friedman's Shoes, had also dropped by to say hello, just in case Dad would need matching shoes.

Max took Dad's measurements and then laid out samples of every color silk for him to peruse. He casually glanced at each color until he spotted a beautiful cream white imported silk square, and pointed it out, "This is it. How long will it take?"

Max paused, then glanced at his calendar. "From two to four weeks," he said. "I'll call you and Mr. Silver when it's ready."

"It would be nice if I could have it by Easter," Dad said, and Max nodded. "Thanks for your help. I really appreciate it. You know, my Counselor here has been mighty kind to me over the years," and then Dad grasped my right hand in his and offered his sincere thanks.

I shall never forget the day—a few weeks later—when I took Dad back to Max for his first fitting. He tried on the suit, with able assistance from Max, his face wreathed in a glowing smile; bright, proud, resplendent. "Counsel, I don't know how to thank you," Dad said to me. "This is the finest thing..."

When I think back on this moment now, I shiver to think that I was watching Daddy King being clothed not only in his Easter finest, but in the same resplendent suit that he would be wearing throughout eternity.

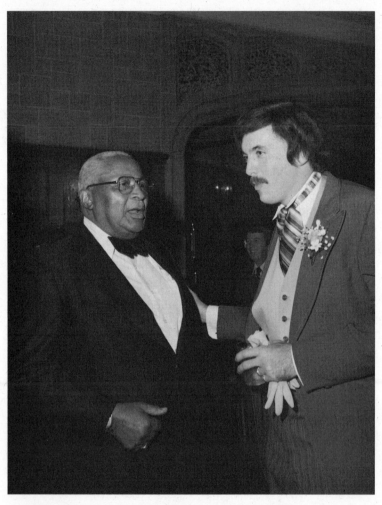

Daddy King and Murray Silver, Jr. at his wedding reception.
Callanwolde Center, Atlanta, GA in November, 1979

Chapter Nine

THE LORD
AIN'T DONE
WITH YOU
YET

———

As early as 1977, Daddy King and I began a weekly ritual of having lunch together. Our schedules permitting, I left my office in the 100 Colony Square Building and picked up Dad promptly at 12:30 pm, then proceeded to the Marriott Hotel on Spring Street, where the hostess always had our table reserved front and center, where guests could view the "Great Man." Frequently other diners requested autographs or to have their photograph made with him. Dad was always patient and kind in accommodating every request.

In time, it wasn't necessary to place an order with the wait staff; Dad always ordered the same thing: New York Strip Steak, medium well, lettuce and tomatoes, sliced onion on the side. The chef knew when to expect us and always set aside the choicest cut. Later in life Dad developed a problem with his teeth and had a difficult time chewing and before cutting into his steak he would prod it with his finger to make certain that it wasn't going to give him any trouble. The chef at the Marriott made sure there would be no complaint.

After lunch, without exception, we stopped by the Silverstar Barber Shop at 181 Auburn Avenue, for Dad's weekly haircut. His barber was Augustus Jordan; no one else was allowed to touch Dad's head. He kept his hair cut short because he complained that when it grew out it itched.

Generally we spent two hours together during these weekly rituals, enjoying various topics of conversation, many of which concerned his family, his church, politics and Atlanta. He kept up with my practice, especially with cases he had referred to me or cases that included racial overtones, and was my liaison with black officers on the police force. He was also aware of my fundraising efforts for the King Center and always appreciative of any favor I might do for the movement both great and small.

I guess one could say that I received a King family education primer, if you please.

Whenever the Silvers gather around the family dinner table and talk turns to the good old days and our unique relationship with the King clan, my oldest son Murray Jr. is fond of relating the story of his first marriage to a lapsed Catholic from Alabama in 1979. The wedding was held at Callanwolde, the ancestral home of the Candler family in Atlanta, the founders of the Coca-Cola Company, and was the first such event outside the Candler clan to be held in the grand manor. Bride and groom were of opposing faiths, and so I imposed upon my dear friend Georgia Supreme Court Justice Charles Weltner to handle the ceremony which my son penned, sounding more like a legal arrangement than a declaration of undying love.

Get the picture: Half of the invitees to this wedding were the Silver clan, which included Coretta Scott King, Daddy King (who was invited to bless the union), and all four of Coretta's children; the other half were the bride's clan from Alabama, who had never been anywhere near people of color and under these circumstances we could only imagine what might ensue when this unlikely gathering converged. Imagine then my great relief when—after the ceremony during which many curious glances were exchanged across the aisle—the bride's family descended upon Coretta and Dad and asked for their autographs.

That is not the end of the story, as my son is want to say. Before the reception in the adjoining dining room was fully underway, Daddy King had grabbed my son and took him to a quiet corner, demanding to know why he had married outside the faith and outside of a church. And for the remainder of the evening, my son tried his best to defend his choice of wife and locale without arguing with Martin Luther King Sr, realizing that nothing he could say was going to get Dad's complete approval. Murray Jr. recalls with a smile that all he had at his wedding reception was half of his cousin's drink and a bite of cake, having spent the rest of the evening being admonished by Daddy King (a photo of which adorns this text).

If you happened to find yourself in the company of Dr. Martin Luther King Sr. at a restaurant, chances are that the owner of the restaurant would be at his personal service. I fondly remember taking Dad to lunch at Pascal's Restaurant on West Hunter Street (renamed Martin Luther King Jr. Blvd.) for a little history and some good food. The Pascal Brothers, James and Robert, had opened their 30-seat lunch counter in 1947, featuring a special recipe Southern fried chicken sandwich, which always recalled the only other great fried chicken I'd ever sampled at Johnny Harris's in Savannah. We were joined at our table by James Pascal, of whom I asked which items on the menu were good.

"Anything on the menu," James said, "but the chicken is really good."

We were then joined by brother Robert, who, pulling up a chair and joining the conversation, took credit for creating the secret recipe for their signature fried chicken dish (and which I understand remains a secret today). Robert's secret for success: "I love to work. No matter how well a task is done, it can be done better, and that is what I set out to do with chicken."

James struck a familiar chord when he stated that he had opened his first business, a shoe shine stand, when he was thirteen years old, which prompted me to interject that my father quit school in the third grade to shine shoes in Savannah. And, like me and my son, the Pascals had also ventured into the music business by opening the Carousel Lounge, an Atlanta jazz mecca that played host to Ramsey Lewis, Aretha Franklin, Lou Rawls, Dizzy Gillespie, and just about every other black touring musician you can name.

Throughout the 1960's, the Pascal brothers had been active in the civil rights movement and their restaurant a meeting place for leaders and strategists. Naturally, the subject of the Robert Felton Moore case came up and, as if on cue, into the restaurant walks Rev. Ralph David Abernathy, the former associate of ML Jr., who acknowledged our having met on the steps of the Camden County Courthouse all those years ago; small world, indeed.

(EDITORIAL NOTE: *Ralph Abernathy was an organizer of the SCLC, and in 1955, when Rosa Parks staged her infamous sit-in, Ralph and ML Jr. organized the bus boycott in Montgomery, Alabama, where Ralph was pastor of the First Baptist Church. An organizer of the March on Washington in 1963, Ralph relocated to Atlanta, where he became pastor of the West Hunter Baptist Church. Along with ML and Bayard Rustin, Ralph was a founder of the SCLC and adopted the motto: "Not one hair of one head of one person should be harmed." Ralph had been at Martin's side in Memphis and had shared Room 336 at the Lorraine Motel the night before the assassination.*)

If you sat around Pascal's Restaurant long enough, you had a very good chance of running into one of Atlanta's best known personalities, Alley Pat. The son of a Baptist preacher, he was one of the city's first black deejays, around the same time that the Pascal brothers were going into the restaurant business. His Christian name was James Patrick, and he got the nickname Alley Pat from frequently suggesting to his listeners that he was about to "get up and go out the alley and drink some beer." His home base was WERD, the first black owned radio station in America, until joining the staff of WAOK in 1954. Alley Pat co-hosted a program with the station's founder, Zenas Sears, a white man with an ear for black music which, at the time, was referred to as Race music. Zenas was responsible for bringing many as yet unknown black artists to the attention of the major record labels, including Piano Red Perryman, who broadcast over WAOK's airwaves from his living room at home (because the station did not have a piano for Red to play in the studio).

I knew all that about Alley Pat, but I knew him better as a local bail bondsman. And I shall never forget the day when Daddy King and I were having lunch at Pascal's with the Pascal brothers, and others gathered around in earshot of our conversation, when Alley Pat entered the establishment and came over to our table to greet everyone. Dad was about to introduce me to Alley Pat when Alley stopped him in mid-introduction: "You don't have to introduce me to Mr. Silver," Alley said. "I've known Mr. Silver since he opened his law office at Colony Square in 1970. And if I ever get into trouble, Lawyer Silver is gonna get me out."

Alley Pat was always quick with a remark. He had interviewed me, Hosea Williams, Jackie Wilson, Maynard Jackson, Don King and just about everybody else of note that came through Atlanta and anywhere near his microphone. Of Pascal's steaks, Alley remarked that they were so juicy "you can cut it with a *thought*." Of Hosea Williams, Alley remarked that he once challenged his reputation as being "Unbought and Unbossed" saying, "Yeah, but you can be rented or leased." And before taking leave of us this day, Alley remarked, "You know, the other day I was talking to a woman who said she was not afraid to go out in her neighborhood after dark even though it has a terrible reputation. She said she didn't need a gun to protect her; Jesus was her protector. And I told her that Jesus ain't no fool: He ain't goin' out in them streets after dark."

And that's what it was like to go to lunch with Daddy King at Pascal's.

Before concluding these memoirs I would be remiss if I did not address a subject that is delicate and controversial, even among King family members, but is never addressed in print and rarely in conversation, that being the strained relationship between Daddy King and his daughter-in-law Coretta. She was born into a family of working class farmers in rural Alabama, and treated to an education that her parents lacked. She received a degree in Voice and Violin at the prestigious New England Conservatory at a time when few black women blessed with her ability had the opportunity to showcase their talent outside the church choir. When ML brought home his intended bride to meet the parents, Dad was opposed to the idea in general, hoping his sons would marry Atlanta women from good families with connections and resources; Coretta, in particular, did not fit the bill. After a serious disagreement, Dad relented and relaxed his opposition to the union and performed the ceremony.

On more than one occasion Dad told me that he actually felt a resentment and bitterness coming from Coretta as a result of his initial attitude toward her. "Coretta held it against me...for some time," he said. Although I did not confirm that impression to Dad, I, too, felt Coretta was not entirely pleased with him based upon casual remarks and her facial expressions whenever we were gathered together. Apparently, healing took a long time and was always in progress without ever being completed.

For the first few years of her marriage to ML, both he and Dad wanted Coretta to focus on family and raising their four children in a good Christian home. Dad's children could quote scripture and read bible stories before going to bed, and the pressure was on Coretta to stay at home and mind the hearth at a time when she desired a more public roll for herself as the wife of a preacher and civil rights leader. Many a time she joined marches and protests arm in arm with her husband. After Martin's death, Coretta began a search for his successor and finding none assumed the role herself. Speaking as her counsel and fellow board member, I think Coretta surprised herself with what she was able to accomplish: a multi-million dollar monument to her husband, the establishment of a national holiday to remember him in perpetuity, and her own place in history as one of the most influential people of her era.

In addition to family matters and affairs of church and state there were, of course, other relaxing topics of conversation for Dad and I to pursue. I once suggested to him that it is interesting to note that most of the leaders of the civil rights movement hailed from the Deep South and that there wasn't a northern liberal among them, which prompted us to make the following list:

Martin Luther King, Sr.	Stockbridge, GA
Martin Luther King, Jr.	Atlanta, GA
Alberta King	Atlanta, GA
Coretta Scott King	Heiberger, AL
Andrew Young	New Orleans, LA
Dr. Bernard Bridges	Atlanta, GA
Rev. Fred Bennette	Atlanta, GA
Leon Hall	Montgomery, AL
Rev. Ralph Abernathy	Linden, AL
John Lewis	Troy, AL

Rev. Joseph Lowery........................Huntsville, AL
Rosa Parks....................................Tuskegee, AL
Barbara Jordan.............................Houston, TX
Rev. Jesse Jackson........................Greenville, SC
Bernard Lee..................................Norfolk, VA
Benjamin Mays.............................Ninety Six, SC
Rev. Fred Shuttlesworth................Mt. Meigs, AL
James Orange...............................Birmingham, AL
James Farmer...............................Marshall, TX
Whitney Young.............................Lincoln Ridge, KY

Of course, the list goes on, but provided much discussion. If some of the names on the list appear unfamiliar to the reader, permit me to remind you of who some of these people were to the civil rights movement:

Dr. Benjamin Mays was one of ML's mentors. The son of former slaves and tenant farmers, Dr. Mays rose to the presidency of Morehouse College, and remained close to ML until his death. "Benny" delivered Martin's eulogy.

Whenever and wherever there was a march or demonstration, you didn't have to look too hard to find James Orange at the forefront leading the procession, shouting orders and giving directions.

James Farmer was a Freedom Rider organizer, one of the Big Four, who along with ML, Whitney Young and Roy Wilkins shaped the civil rights movement.

John Lewis survived a vicious attack during the Selma-to-Montgomery march and later became a member of the US House of Representatives from Georgia.

Bernard Lee was Martin's personal assistant and travel companion from the early days of the movement. A member of the inner circle, Bernard shielded ML from reporters and was adored for his sense of humor. He was considered to be indispensable to the movement, and ML made Bernard's travel expenses a prerequisite for accepting invitations; that Bernard was with Martin in Memphis when he was assassinated is typically overlooked by most accounts. I had the pleasure of meeting Bernard for the first time during the Robert Felton Moore trial in 1966.

I had met all of the individuals mentioned in the above list and had shared experiences with many of them. Dad's ability to remember each and their contributions always fascinated me. I could listen to him endlessly whenever he reflected on the past.

Every now and then Dad and I talked about religion. God was the major force in his life, and his heritage had been religious: "...and now abideth faith, hope, charity, these three; but the greatest of these is charity." Dad often referred to the passage from St. Matthew, "Inasmuch as ye have done it unto one of the least of these my brethren, ye have done it unto me." When talk turned to his grandchildren, Dexter and MLIII, why then did they not pursue the ministry? And Dad would reply, "For many are called, but few are chosen," and declined to elaborate. However, it seemed to me that he would have been especially pleased had his namesake decided to follow in the footsteps of his predecessors. The tone of Dad's voice changed whenever he referred to Marty, and one of Dad's last requests was that I would always remain close to Marty. I further conclude that of his grandchildren Marty favored Dad most in appearance.

What was it that drove Martin Luther King, Sr.? I vividly recall his answer to that question, as it was posed to him by my oldest son: "You use what you have over the years, just like you do, but God put me in a position to be used." He later elaborated on the topic during one of our luncheons: "The spirit of the Lord is upon me because He anointed me to preach the gospel to the poor. We are to do something for the down trodden, broken hearted, the unemployed, the captive, blind, bruised..." Interrupting, "Sounds like you might've used that once or twice before in sermons?" Smiling, Dad nodded in agreement.

Intelligence plus character is how I remember ML Sr.

In preparing these brief remarks I discussed Dad with his granddaughter, Alveda King. In response to my question, "How would you describe Dad's major characteristics or distinguishing traits?" she replied, without hesitating, "In two words: compassion and strength."

I also remember, with a smile, the assessment of Daddy King by Jewel Futch, who had been the sheriff of Lowndes County, GA, from 1954-64, and past president of the Georgia Sheriff's Association. Jewel remembered Dad most favorably, saying, "I couldn't make up my mind whether he was a Good Ol' Big Un or a Big Ol' Good Un."

As for the Sweet Auburn community at large, most remember Daddy King for his Sunday services at Ebenezer, which were always special. Beautiful music, choir, colorful, spiritually uplifting; you did not have to be Southern Baptist to appreciate what transpired during all those celebrations. Clothed in his pastoral splendor, Dad conducted his sermons—oft quoted—in a highly energized, electric oratory that were often punctuated by choruses of "Amen" or "Tell it" from the pews. I confess, on several occasions, from my point of observation on the back row, I was moved to the point of being ready to jump and shout "Amen, Dad, Amen!"

Without question, Martin Luther King, Sr. had a delivery every bit as powerful as his illustrious son, although not as widely broadcast. And I admit here, for the first time, Dad's profound influence over my own oratorical skills as a defense lawyer, who was once described by Time magazine as a "fire breather."

The act of setting down these memoirs has been an act of pure inspiration and joy. Perhaps it is many stories in one, yet all one story really. I think of it as a gallant story of the irrepressible spirit of a giant of a man. What is gallantry? I define it as dashing courage, heroic bravery, high spirited defiance in the face of danger. My own Daddy often said to me, "It is no disgrace in getting knocked down; the disgrace is lying there."

Of all the things Daddy King ever said to me, the words I remember most and will continue to remember until my dying day was said to me at one of the most beleaguered points in my professional career, when I exhausted myself in representing several prominent members of the "Mob" and had gained an excessive amount of publicity resulting in an investigation into my affairs by the Alphabet Boys: the FBI, CIA and IRS. Agents were sitting on my doorstep, tailing me in unmarked cars, tapping my phones. Having practically no one else in which to confide my frustration but Dad, he remarked, "One thing is for certain: they can't eat you!"

I shall also remember always his admonition to me at the conclusion of many of our telephone calls, "Counselor, the Lord ain't done with you yet! Keep on keepin' on!"

My friend Damon Runyon, the great news reporter and writer of short stories about the glory days on Broadway, used to say, "There is a Tavern at the End of the Road, where we shall all meet again, renew our deep friendships and swap yarns once more as we have done in so many places and at so many times around the globe and over the years. Between innings, between halves, between rounds, between sprints, waiting for juries, or for election returns, or reports from the FBI, at Dempsey's, Fisherman's Wharf, and Brown Hotel." To that I would add Johnny Harris Restaurant in Savannah, where I know I have friends waiting for me in that tavern, with whom I have made a date all too soon. The most exciting aspect to this book is that all these friends, these remarkable men and women, these great Americans, the great, near great and not so great, commoners and Kings, will walk with me in remembrance as clear as the events themselves all the days of my life.

On November 11, 1984, that gallant heart stopped beating. I stood in line with thousands of others to pay final respects, as the casket was delivered to Morehouse College at 12:49 pm. Hugh Gloster, the school's president, approached me and shared the recollection that "he was known as 'Dad' by many students, who consulted him about religion, academic and financial matters," and as I approached the casket a reporter from a local television station asked me for a few comments. "He was a father to me," I said. "I consulted him when I needed help, and I needed it frequently. He offered me a great deal of consolation, and of all the people I have known, he would rank second or third closest to me."

I was also reminded of a time when, shortly after Alberta's death, I asked Dad, "Considering the enormous tragedies that you have endured, how do you find the strength to keep on keepin' on?"

To which Dad replied, "You know, Counsel, I'm tired, but I will keep on going. I love preaching. I have a deep faith in God, and in the power of love. Now I want you to know that I am not dyin' to get home; I'm gonna go to sleep and when I wake up, I'll be home."

Weeks passed, and I visited his grave site to find the headstone shared with his beloved Bunch filled in:

THE REV. MARTIN LUTHER KING, SR.

"DADDY" KING

DEC. 19, 1899

NOV. 11, 1984

I LOVE EVERYONE

STILL IN BUSINESS, JUST MOVED UPSTAIRS

...a final, well said tribute. And, in conclusion, I can think of no better epitaph for this great American religious and civil rights leader: "May it ring down from the mountain tops and fill the valleys all over the world, that we are all in this together, and white, black, yellow and red, shout and regale, I CANNOT HATE ANY MAN!"

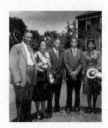

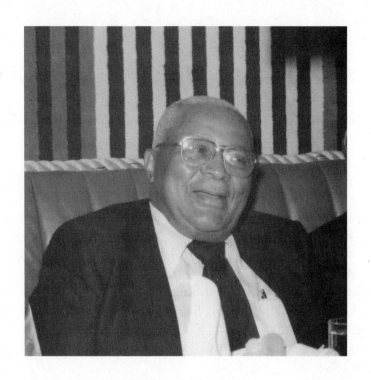

AFTERWORD

Fred Bennette died on March 5, 1994, at age 65. Although few had gathered around to help him during his final illness, hundreds of former civil rights marchers, community leaders and activists packed Ebenezer Baptist Church on March 11th to say goodbye. Joseph Lowery, President of SCLC, said a few words, Andrew Young said a few words, Coretta Scott King spoke in Bennette's behalf, as well as Dr. Bernard Bridges, but the eulogy was left to me, as was Bennette's final request "that his lawyer say whatever needed to be said."

I had visited Bennette every day in the hospital not only out of respect but because he complained to me that "they're not treating me right." Bennette was running up a telephone bill that looked like the national debt and the hospital cut off his phone when they were instructed by Bennette's insurance provider that they weren't going to cover the charges. Bennette without a phone was like a man without a head; he couldn't live without being in constant contact with those that kept him in his customary loop. Bennette complained to his doctor and every nurse in the unit that he was going to get his lawyer to sue them if they did not restore his phone service. He threatened to call Andy Young and when that didn't work, he threatened to have the hospital picketed. And when that didn't work, he called me in on the case. His telephone privileges were restored.

To visit a sick friend in the hospital is to summon the strength to keep smiling and present a cheerful countenance, even when dealing with farewells. I didn't want to add to Bennette's burdens by sitting around and complaining or allowing him to complain, preferring to recall some of the good times we had together. I was reminded, in particular, of a wonderful day we had spent together back in 1976, shortly after Jimmy Carter had announced his candidacy for president and Rev. Bennette called on me to help him sound the call to action among the black community. He had called me on a late Friday afternoon and told me he would drop by my house early on Saturday morning to show me his new car, but his real reason was to get me to go with him to meet a group of black preachers in Ft. Valley.

Bennette arrived at my house at 9:30 sharp—not CPT (Colored People's Time)—with an O'Jay's tape blaring from his sound system, and we then proceeded along the interstate in a southerly direction.

"You ever been to McDonough?" Bennette asked me.

"Why, yes, as a matter of fact, I've tried four cases there. I know everybody over to the courthouse. You know, I'm the only lawyer in Georgia history to have tried cases in every one of her 159 counties."

"Oh? Well, how many preachers do you know?" Bennette asked.

"None."

"Then we gonna fix that," he said, and steered toward Cleveland Chapel AME, where we were greeted by her pastor and ten other ministers.

After introductions were made and pleasantries exchanged, Bennette got down to business: "We are here to meet you in hopes that we can get you to join us in getting our governor elected president. Daddy King is on board and Andy Young is on board. We need you to get folks registered and get out the vote."

And the ministers wasted no time in getting right down to business: "That's all well and good, Reverend Bennette, but who will we look to? You know, it's easy to get things started, but it's hard to keep going. We all pastor small churches: one hundred, two hundred, no more than four hundred members, mostly farmers and wage earners. Are any expenses involved?"

At that point, Bennette looked at me, saying, "My lawyer can tell you about that..." although I was taken completely by surprise. I hardly knew what to say. My dear friend had not alerted me to the fact that I would be called upon to say a few words about fundraising.

"I'm here at the invitation of Reverend Bennette, gentlemen. I have known Jimmy Carter since before he was elected Governor of Georgia. I believe him to be a good Christian, an honest, hard working farmer who has had a hard row to hoe and has an even harder one in running for president. Money is being raised. It will take time, but with your help, I feel like all expenses will be met."

There was a certain amount of hesitation in the room as I had stopped short of explaining exactly how much would be available and how soon, but it was only because I had no clue as to the answer to either question. The ministers looked at me and concluded that I had just made some sort of promise, and Bennette saw an opportunity to make a clean getaway before I was pressed for details. We shook hands all around and patted each other on the back and headed for Bennette's car. With a little luck, I thought I might be able to get home in time to spend the afternoon with my family; Bennette had made other plans.

Our next stop was Friendship AME Church on Highway 16 in East Jackson. It was getting near lunch time and I suggested that we stop for a bite to eat first, but Bennette told me that the church members were expecting us to break bread with them in their fellowship hall. Apparently, Bennette was aware of all sorts of details that he had not told me about. We were met by a welcoming committee of eighteen smiling faces who served up a bountiful repast of fried chicken and mashed potatoes, collard greens, salad, jello, sweet tea, rolls and butter. I must admit it was finger lickin' good.

Following lunch, the presentation went as it had gone before in McDonough, at the end of which I told Bennette, "If we keep this up, we gonna be good advocates for the Peanut Man."

Macon, Warner Robbins, and Ft. Valley followed before the long day was done. Mayors of the last two were included. Dinner was offered by the deacons of St. Paul's AME in Macon, where Pastor Mallory presided over a supper of—you guessed it: fried chicken, etc.

"At least we ate good that day," Bennette interrupted me to say.

"We did. And do you remember what you said to me when we got home?"

Bennette shook his head and smiled. "I thanked you for doing me the favor, but I told you I didn't have any money to pay for favors..."

"And I said I don't charge for them."

"My lawyer," Bennette said, extending his hand, just as he did on that pleasant evening all those years ago.

The thought occurred to me that Bennette still had a lot of living to do and that his insistence that he stay in touch by telephone was a good indication that he would be going home from the hospital, but the Lord had other plans.

"Fred Bennette had a love affair with the SCLC and the movement," said Rev. Lowery, at Bennette's funeral. "He married the movement. He was protective of its leaders and would defend them with his life. He was straightforward and believed in telling it like it is."

Andy Young recalled the incident at the rally for the Freedom Riders in Montgomery, when a bomb was hurled at Martin Luther King, Jr. "Bennette knocked everybody out of harm's way. He never hesitated; he picked up the bomb and threw it away just seconds before it detonated. And then it was left to Mrs. King to remind the mourners that even in the last hours of his final illness Bennette was busy organizing her security detail for an out-of-town engagement. He remained Chief of Security to the King family and the Center, affectionately known as "The Commandant," until his last breath.

It was then left up to me to put a fine point on the life and sacrifices of Fred Bennette in his eulogy. I had come prepared to do the job equipped with my old family bible, from which I was to read a couple of pertinent passages, but as I entered the church and was greeted by Andy Young and Mrs. King, Joe Lowery spotted the Good Book and said, "You're not gonna preach to us, are you, Murray? Please, leave the drivin' to us!" So I set the bible aside as I began my farewell, and I vividly recall that it went something like this:

"Fred Bennette was truly a man...a real man...a man's man. He was honest, reliable, forthright, opinionative, outspoken. I never heard him curse, use profanity or criticize another; if he didn't like you, he would tell you, but he wouldn't talk behind your back. He was as big as one of the old oak trees that Daddy King always liked to talk about: he was brave and feared no man; a teacher who had a wonderful way with children. He was truly a man for all seasons. And what was this giant of a man to me? He was my friend for over 27 years. And what is a friend? I'll tell you: A friend is a person with whom you dare to be yourself. He seems to ask you to put on nothing, only to be what you really are. When you are with him, you do not have to be on guard. You can say what you think, so long as it is genuinely you. With him you breathe freely—you can state your little vanities and envies and absurdities, and in opening up to him, they are dissolved in the ocean of his loyalty. He understands—you can weep with him, laugh with him, pray with him; through and underneath it all he sees, knows and loves you. A friend, I repeat, is one whom you dare to be yourself. And so my Heavenly Father, I commend to you my dear friend. Well done, thou good and faithful servant. Let the words of my mouth and the meditation of my heart be acceptable before thee, O Lord, my Rock and my Redeemer."

With the passing of Daddy King and Fred Bennette and ultimately with the death of Coretta Scott King, the torch has been passed to a new generation, namely the children of ML Jr. and Coretta—one of whom, Yolanda, has also passed—and the children of Christine King and Isaac Farris. It is with deep regret and a keen sense of personal loss to note that the passing of the torch has involved a few notable slips, resulting in legal disputes among siblings over the intellectual property rights of their parents. In my customary role as counsel to the King family I have—from my porch rocking chair at the beach—endeavored to be of help in mending these rifts and in the spirit expected of me by Daddy King, had he been here to guide us all through it.

I mention the foregoing if for no other reason than to tell you this:

At a time when Dexter Scott King was assuming the leadership of the King Center from his mother, his cousin Isaac Farris, Jr. replaced Coretta as Chief Operating Officer. Isaac had graduated from Morehouse, where he majored in Political Science. I had known him since birth, and remember as a child he was always in attendance at the joint birthday parties held for my wife Barbara and Coretta on April 27. As an adult I often crossed paths with Isaac during the campaign to get Walter Mondale elected president in 1984, and later when he managed Andy Young's campaign for mayor of Atlanta. Isaac married Jackie White, who had been in the ranks of Young for Congress, and thereafter was one of Andy's trusted friends and advisors.

Andy Young was elected to the first of two terms as mayor of Atlanta in 1981. I had campaigned for him, sponsored fundraisers, luncheons and concerts, and shortly after taking office I received a telephone call from Jackie Farris, who had called to say that Andy wanted to do something in recognition of all that I had done for him. I responded, "Jackie, I do not know one thing that Andy can do for me. I've got a great trial practice and I really don't need anything."

The following day Jackie called to ask for an appointment to see me in person, at which he said rather forcefully that "Andy will not accept your answer. He wants to appoint you Judge of Municipal Court. He insists."

Two weeks later, Murray M. Silver was appointed Judge, Municipal Court of Atlanta, and served with distinction for eight years, and resigned after filing a formal complaint about the collection procedures of traffic fines implemented during the Bill Campbell administration which followed Andy's tenure and ended in the arrest, trial and imprisonment of Mayor Campbell.

Retrospection

Daddy King "moved upstairs" on November 11, 1984. It is difficult for me to realize that he has been gone for almost 25 years. Let's look back at events that have taken place, bearing in mind the famous people that have the whole earth as their memorial. Daddy King stated to me on more than one occasion, "You can't give up in life. If you lose hope, you lose the vitality that keeps life moving. You lose that courage to be, that quality that helps you go on in spite of it all."

At the outset, I observed, "The single most important impression I want to leave the reader with is that history has not paid Martin Luther King Sr. his due. If the civil rights movement had a father, it was Daddy King, in the same way that he was father to his son."

Dexter Scott King, born January 30, 1961, replaced his mother as CEO of the King Center in Atlanta, and is presently working on a book about her life.

Rev. Bernice Albertine King, born March 28, 1963, is the spiritual keeper of her father's and grandfather's legacy as pastor at New Birth Missionary Baptist Church in Atlanta. A powerful motivational speaker, Bunny often refers to her grandfather in her sermons and carries on his *Somebodiness* theme.

Yolanda Denise King, born November 17, 1955, pursued her grandfather's and father's dream of racial harmony as a dramatic actor and motivational speaker until her untimely death in May 2007, less than 18 months following the death of her mother.

Coretta Scott King, founder of the King Center in Atlanta, died on January 30, 2006, after a lifetime of accomplishments in her own right, including championing her husband's birthday as a national holiday and the perpetual preservation of his intellectual properties.

Christine King Farris, the eldest and only living child of Daddy King, is an associate professor at Spelman College, author of several books, public speaker, and occupies many roles at the King Center, NAACP, and SCLC. Her son Isaac Newton Farris Jr. currently serves as CEO of the King Center.

Martin Luther King III, born October 23, 1957, attended Morehouse College, in the tradition of his forefathers, and rose in the ranks from community activist to the presidency of the SCLC, an organization founded by his father. An eloquent, passionate speaker who takes strong positions on civil rights, he has made a name for himself as an international leader, having spoken on behalf of Sen. Barack Obama at the Democratic National Convention in 2008, and as founder of Realizing the Dream. His daughter, Yolanda Renee King, named in honor of his late sister, is the first grandchild of Martin Luther King Jr and Coretta Scott King.

On January 1, 1900, there was only one African-American member of the US Congress. One hundred years later, there were 39 black representatives, including 14 women, all of whom owe a debt of gratitude to Daddy

King. To look back at the "Black Church" over the past one hundred years is to recall some of the most important moments in history: the fight for education, the battle for civil rights, the quest for women's rights—the church was more than just a place of worship, it was a school, theatre, community center, meeting place, political engine, and in each category Daddy King was the vanguard, at the forefront of the movement, mounting the charge.

Without him, it would have been a different century in America.

Postscript

As I travel about making speeches to schools, civic groups and church meetings, it has become increasingly clear to me that the black youth of today do not know the history of their people. They don't know where they've been and they don't know where they're going. They know Oprah, Michael Jordan, and Beyonce, but draw a blank on Harry Belafonte, Willie Mays, and Paul Robeson. In order for black America to move forward, history must be remembered and recalled.

In pursuit of this argument, I cite Sen. Barack Obama, on November 13, 2006, at the groundbreaking ceremony of the Martin Luther King Jr. National Memorial: "My children might ask why is this monument here, what did this man do? My response is: He gave his life serving others, he tried to love *somebody*." Well, the speaker, I respectfully submit, could've told it like it was: Obama should have given Daddy King credit for the expression and he should've gotten it right: Somebodiness was a subject that Daddy King often preached and taught it to his children and grandchildren, and then the speaker should've stated it correctly: It wasn't that Martin "tried to love somebody," he tried to love everybody!

My point is further advanced by none other than

Christine King Farris, in an interview with Tom Brokaw, televised nationally on Nov. 12, 2008, in which Brokaw inquired, "Why is it that young people know Chris Rock but not your brother?" Christine replied: "Young people don't know. They don't know how a black person was elected to lead us. They need to hear it as Daddy King preached, 'Make it plain.'"

I hope that this book sheds light on my dear friend, a giant of a man, "The Father of the Civil Rights Movement in America."

I made it plain.

I rest my case.

INDEX

About the Author

Murray M. Silver, Esq., Judge, was born in Savannah, Georgia on October 15, 1929, to Catherine Mendel and Wolfe W. Silver. Attended Charles Ellis Elementary School, Richard Arnold Junior High School and Benedictine Military School, graduating in 1947. Upon graduating from Armstrong Junior College in 1949, entered the University of Georgia School of Law in September of that year. His studies were interrupted when he was called to active duty in the "Mighty Eighth" United States Air Force during the Korean War. Graduated from Law School and admitted to practice in October, 1953, entered private practice with offices in Savannah, Ga.

He was President Benedictine's class of 1947; "Most Outstanding Sophomore," A.J.C; Chancellor of Tau Epsilon Phi Fraternity, Law School Honor Court, President of B'nai B'rith; Founder of Savannah Little League Baseball, Manager and Coach, winning City Championship twice.

Founder of Savannah Legal Aid Society and named to "Who's Who in American Law," 1978; Appointed General Counsel, Georgia Department of Labor in 1967, served three years with distinction, returned to private practice in Atlanta, Ga. Member of the Georgia Bar 44 years, admitted to practice in the United States Supreme Court, Court of Appeals; 10 U. S. District Courts. Appointed Judge, Municipal Court of Atlanta by Mayor Andrew J. Young, Jr., served eight years with distinction. A prominent trial lawyer, handling over 3,000 cases in 42 states, the District of Columbia, Argentina, England, Bahamas, Jamaica, Antigua. His clients came from all walks of life, including Dr. William B. Shockley, Nobel Laureate; Sports stars, Entertainers, five "Godfathers," and "The World's Biggest Drug Trafficker." Retired, October 31, 1997.

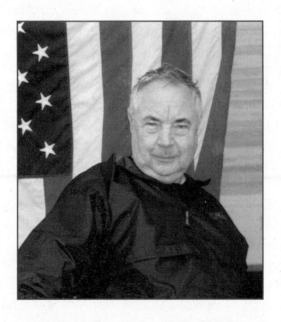

Visit **www.DaddyKingBook.com** for Judge Murray M. Silver's book tour, speaking engagements and more.